IT DOESN'T HAVE TO BE LIKE THIS

FROM HOPELESS TO HOPEFUL

JARED M. LANCE

Disclaimer

All the material contained in this book is provided for educational and informational purposes only.

No responsibility can be taken for any results or outcomes resulting from the use of this material.

ACKNOWLEDGMENTS

My dad, Larry Lance - you taught me faith and how without it, we will be lost. You saved my life and to you, I owe the world.

My mom, Becky Lance – you showed me love during the darkest times when I felt all alone, and for that, I love you even more.

My brother, Justin Lance – you inspired me with hope for a better future. You and your beautiful wife, Heather Lance, gave me a nephew, Easton Lance, with whom I can now create a secret handshake.

My family in Michigan, thanks for always loving me and encouraging me along the way.

To my friends and mentors: Matt Hammons, Joe Pasquali, Seth Lochmueller, Nicholas Weaver, Abrielle Haver, Kelly Cochran, Matt Rayls, Andrew Stout, Chris Todia, Ryan Lough, Phil Marquell, Joshua Dapkus, Bobby Cortez, JJ Gorena II, Eric Defreeuw, Nathan Carden, Angel Flores, Dave Long, Ryan & Kacie Miller, Sarah Bradbury, Lamonte Rhoades, Luther Whitfield, Phil Johnson, Jim Posey, Josh VonGunten, Anthony Opliger, thank you for being in my life and giving me the strength to keep going.

Special thanks to my coworkers at Parkview Health and Namaste Health for giving me an opportunity to work for such amazing organizations.

To everyone who has supported me through this journey, you are loved. I am so incredibly thankful that I get to share this story. Thank you and God bless!

TABLE OF CONTENTS

INTRODUCTION

This book is written to share, connect and empathize on a relatable level with individuals who feel depressed, frustrated and melancholic through firsthand experiences, facts, and testimonies on various subjects not limited to mental health, selflessness, faith, loneliness, and healthy habits.

We have all felt alone, hopeless, or defeated at times. That sense of disappointment or failure does not have to weigh us down. Encouraging someone else, giving them hope, and helping them to stay on their feet are some of the greatest feelings we can ever experience. No matter what has happened or presently happening in your life, do not lose hope for better days. Do not EVER give up.

Always remember that this life is a blessing—never forget that. If we have taken a breath on this planet, then we have a story to tell. The problem with us, however, is that the embarrassment of our mistakes often beclouds our vision and prevents us from seeking the help that we need to live a better and more fulfilling life. We judge ourselves too harshly and conclude that we're inadequate and don't deserve help or love. The good news is that, now, I am able to share my story with people and offer the help I once needed so desperately. I would never ever want to lose someone to suicide when it is completely avoidable.

Can we be bold and make a difference in someone's life today? Absolutely Yes! Maybe there is someone we are already considering reaching out to. Maybe we're the ones who need to speak up and talk. Don't be ashamed of your story. It will inspire others.

Having the ability to relate to mental illness was also a key component in writing this book. I would be the first to admit that I was judgmental about mental illness ab initio, ignorant of the reasons life turned out sour for others when it seemed so beautiful. As my hypocrisy came full circle, I lapsed into circumstantial depression and quickly became aware of how incredibly important it is to address mental health.

My main purpose in writing this book is to help you become more conscious and intentional about the decisions you make and how you live your life. This awareness came from my past failures and poor decisions. Rather than complaining and pointing fingers, I wanted to take the initiative to try to be the helper. There is no right or wrong answer when it comes to choosing priorities. The main idea is to take control by doing the right thing for the people you encounter every day. Help them live better lives; encourage them to be different and excited about their future. Encourage them to have fun and cherish every single moment of their lives.

Come with me now on this journey from hopeless to hopeful.

Shall we?

CHAPTER 1
JUMPER

"There are far, far better things ahead than anything we leave behind."
– C.S. Lewis

It was a beautiful Monday morning, but my mind didn't share in any of that beauty. I was desperate. I felt as if I had wasted most of the past 10 years on the wrong path.

I had taken many wrong actions and was suffering the consequences. Previously I had broken my ankle playing basketball with friends. After I had a second surgery on this ankle, I began taking Lorazepam and Hydrocodone to deal with the pain. I got addicted to the feeling of numbness and release from the pressures of life. Once I continued to take the medications for a couple of months, I started to lose myself. I had no real feelings toward anything or anyone. I spent weeks lying on a couch wishing life would get better. However, nothing comes easy and no magic pill could fix my suffering. My awareness for making smart decisions was gone. At least that is what I told myself as I continued to spin my life into a disaster.

I was simply going through the motions and trying to have as much fun as possible in between all the sadness and despair. I hopped in my Volkswagen GTI and headed out of my apartment complex down 30th

Street in Colorado Springs, Colorado. I passed Garden of the Gods, the majestic deep-red rock formations and marveled at Pikes Peak in the background. I continued my drive until I got to Cheyenne Canyon, where Mount Cutler is located.

I parked the car, put on my headphones, laced up my shoes, and started the short hike up the trail. It was slightly less than a mile to the top, but for me, it was just the perfect little trail to hike. I had been struggling with rehabbing from my second ankle surgery, so anything longer than this, and I probably would have been pushing it too much. I remember listening to the letter Paul wrote to the Galatians on the way up the trail. It shook me—he was so frustrated that everyone had lost focus on Jesus. Paul made it simple: Trust in Christ, not in the law. As we are saved by faith, so we must walk by faith. Galatians 5:1 says, "It is for freedom that Christ has set us free. Stand firm, then, and do not let yourselves be burdened again by a yoke of slavery." I took the last five minutes walking to reflect on what I had just heard. I felt like a part of this statistic Paul had mentioned. I had strayed from God's path. Once I got to the top, I decided to call my father.

I made it to the top of the rock overlooking the immaculate western Colorado sky as the phone rang a few times. He answered with his classic, "Hey Jared!" This was always how we started our phone calls, and it made me laugh every single time. I responded with "Hey Larry!" in a similarly goofy tone. We chatted for a few minutes as I struggled to tell him the truth. No matter how much I tried, I couldn't bring myself to own up and tell my old man that my life was a mess. I was sweating and breathing heavily, and he could tell something was seriously wrong. The truth was that I needed money, I needed help, and I needed peace and reassurance. I needed answers, but all I had were questions masked with lies. Our brief conversation about my recent stock trading venture came to an end. I had again managed to hide my troubles behind a flippant discussion. My father played along and answered me casually too, but I was sure he saw beyond my goofiness and knew I was unhappy deep down. He simply let it slide because he didn't want to embarrass me by pushing too hard.

I thought about how he had overcome mentally, emotionally, and physically abusive parents, and how he got to where he is today. This contributed to the sinking feeling I felt. I hadn't gone through half of the challenges my father had overcome, yet, here was I unable to do anything meaningful with my life. I felt like a waste of time, space, and God's grace. I didn't feel the need to keep up with the charade and continue living a lie any longer. Looking down from the dizzying height of Mount Cutler, it occurred to me that this would be a good time to end it all for good. I began to contemplate suicide. There were not many clouds in the sky at this point of the day, but my head was certainly cloudy. Negativity had resided in my brain for so many months that I honestly felt suicide was the best solution. At that moment, I was a complete monster.

My heart was pounding in my chest. The pain was unbearable, and I wasn't willing to endure it any longer. I had experienced plenty of physical pain before: broken collarbones, broken ankle, surgeries, a hernia, car crashes, and multiple concussions. And I can confidently tell you that physical pain does not even come close to emotional pain in intensity. The devil was winning the battle, and I was letting it happen. I felt the same rush one gets from skydiving or bungee jumping. There was a part of me that wanted it to happen while the other part wasn't ready to go just yet. On one side, I was done with life, I'd had enough and just wanted to end it all. Yet, at the same time, I could feel the wind in my face and see the shining sun and I didn't feel like giving those things up.The devil was on one shoulder, and an angel was on the other. As I leaned over the ledge, adrenaline kicked in, and I began gasping for air. I was having an out–of-body experience. I couldn't hear anything. For the first time in my life, I felt as if I had completely lost control. I covered my eyes for a second and tried to take a deep breath. I was ready to jump, ready to say goodbye to it all, ready for the sadness to go away. I closed my eyes and imagined what it would feel like to fall hundreds of feet to my death. I pictured it; the mess and the loss, the sick and disgusting leap that would wreck my bones and body as well as the emotions of the many people I loved. The only thought in my brain at the time was, can I jump off? Can I die? Can I actually commit suicide?

For whatever reason, that strong urge to jump as well as the adrenaline rush subsided momentarily. My hearing returned, and I could breathe properly again. As I opened my eyes to see the beautiful mountain edges, I had a small epiphany. I was surrounded by pure silence, and I knew I was just missing the point. It was so peaceful outside. I realized that all the sadness, despair and emotional turmoil I felt was only within me. Out there, it was peaceful and calm, even beautiful. It occurred to me that taking that leap would only be my loss. I would jump and die, yet these breathtaking rocks would remain there. The sun would still rise the next day. The beautiful birds in the sky would still chirp and make their sonorous sounds. Even the people who loved me would mourn, some for a short time, some for a long time. But eventually, they would get over me and life would continue for them as usual. Then, out of nowhere, the thought hit me like a ton of bricks; LIFE IS NOT JUST ABOUT ME, THERE'S FAR MORE! I sat there for 30 to 45 minutes knowing suicide was not the answer. I was just a small part of a huge universe created by an even bigger force and killing myself would really not change anything. I would read through some Proverbs, say a prayer, sit in silence, and just listen. I took some time with God and asked a whole bunch of questions. I asked questions about life. About why I made so many poor decisions. Why was I so unhappy? Why do I lie to everyone? Why did I lose my passion for life? These questions kept tumbling through my mind and I wondered how I had missed the point all this while and gotten so tangled up in my sordid little life.

I spent a lot of time on that mountain trying to sort through the tangle of emotions I felt. After the epiphany, I was sure suicide wasn't the best step to take. So instead of jumping, I decided to try to troubleshoot my life and come up with logical solutions. I knew I needed to get help, I needed to stop trading stocks, and I needed to turn my life around completely. My brain was dead, and I could barely process any of the terrible decisions I was making. This was the reason why I was so depressed, and I knew I had to tackle this too. At least I had made one right decision by choosing not to jump, I thought that was a good starting point. There were so many problems I had never addressed with my friends and family that it almost felt too late. I had completely ignored facing the facts and just being honest with people.

After almost an hour of sitting and thinking in silence, I noticed someone coming up the trail. It was a young lady and her dog. They both sat about 50 yards or so from me, in a similar position on a rock overlooking the ledge. The difference was she looked happy, as if she were enjoying her life to the fullest. For a minute I felt hopeful. I thought, *wow, I am taking this life for granted. I spend so much time complaining about my own pain, that I completely ignore everyone and everything else in the world.*

After mulling over the issue for so long, I knew what I had to do next, and it was not going to be pretty, but it was necessary. Knowing isn't difficult, it's doing; taking action, that's the hard part. I had been a compulsive liar most of my life. I was always afraid to tell the truth, I feared letting people see beyond the façade I put up and into my soul. I wasn't sure that anyone would be willing to accept me for who I was. I was unsure who would be there at the end to help me become the man God created me to be. I thought about my loved ones and how this would affect them. As the confessions came pouring out to friends and family, change was imminent. It was time to move back home and start my life over.

We all make the mistake of adopting temporary fixes and seeing them as permanent solutions. In my case, it was my addiction to pills, for others it may be gambling or watching pornography. And when these quick fixes don't bring the long-term satisfaction they expect, they don't see the point any longer, and then they just jump. My faith in God ultimately kept me from jumping, but how sickening to even be that close! Some people lose touch with what truly matters in life, and they just snap.

Many people are not as fortunate as I was, and some don't get the chance to start over. Many, unlike myself, don't have family or a place to move back to. I finally saw how lucky I was to be able to have support from friends and family. I got my wakeup call though, and it was time to stop complaining and start being thankful for everything. I knew I had been deceitful. I had been a bad son and a bad friend. I kept asking questions like, why am I doing this? Why am I doing this to myself? The people around me deserved a better friend and family member. Then I realized God loved me and would forgive me for all of this, if I would just step back from the ledge. From that day forward, I could start over and choose the right path. I was blown away by that thought. I had never truly had a moment where I needed to even consider starting over.

I was such an unthankful child! I kept fighting the thoughts of regret and missing out. I wanted to be back in San Antonio, I wanted to stay in Colorado Springs, and I kept living in a moment that no longer existed.

The fact is, I barely took the time to enjoy living in those moments anyway, because I was not mentally stable. Everything was so fleeting. From going to see my beloved Detroit Tigers play in different cities across the country, to visiting various national parks, to seeing my favorite bands perform— all of the pleasure that came with doing those things just vanished. The difference was that I was pleasure seeking, for myself, and I was not joyful seeking. This is why I continue to say that temporary satisfaction will never be a permanent fixture for our brokenness. There is no drug, no drink, no concert, no baseball game or vacation that will ever give us what faith, hope, and love can. My selfish decisions were a huge detriment to my relationships, my friendships, and my happiness. Thank God I got a second chance to start over.

After that moment of truth on the rock, it was time for the trip back to Indiana to be with my family for a week or so and process all the previous events. My father and I flew back to Colorado a few days later to start packing. It took us most of the day to pack away everything in a U-Haul truck with my Volkswagen towed on the back. There were some heavy emotions that went with packing my entire life into a 15-foot box truck. I felt myself hitting an all-time low, this was me and all I had. Everything that belonged to me and defined me conveniently fit in a truck that was not even up to half of some people's homes. I felt tears burning at the back of my eyes, but I pushed them back.

As we started the drive through Kansas, out of nowhere, a deer decided to cross the road. I heard a loud scream, "Jared!!!" Before I could even react, I smashed that deer going about 60mph. My night vision was not the greatest, and my brain was all out of whack. Just before the deer strayed into the vehicle's path, we had been talking about how amazing the blood orange moon looked. My dad had suggested to me, about five minutes before that we should pull over and take a picture of it. He mentioned that he wanted to send a picture of the moon to my mom. I felt he was being unnecessarily sentimental and disagreed, saying we didn't have time to waste. How ironic? Or did God truly give me a sign that I neglected? The answer is obvious now: My neglect once again led to disaster. I was being selfish again; I wasn't considerate of how much my mom would have appreciated that little act of love and affection.

We got out to assess the damage and I began to laugh; my dad did too.

God certainly has a unique sense of humor. This was the confirmation that I was at the beginning of the journey towards a fresh start. I knew that this was it, the rock bottom I needed to hit so I could bounce back. There was not even a moment that I asked the question, "How could this happen to me?" I knew this was the plan all along. Because now I would actually pay attention and fix my mistakes. As cliché as it is, everything happens for a reason. Some of us need some crazy events to happen to make us realize that life is precious.

Once you have your version of the hitting-a-deer-in-Kansas-moment, you'll know that life could always be worse. Deep down I knew holding on to the past was just like driving on an uncompleted bridge that led to nowhere. You would end up crashing into a river or a canyon.

It's pretty simple: If we lose touch with ourselves, evil grabs hold. If we lose the balance that is needed in life to maintain happy and healthy relationships, evil starts to take over. If we have no one holding us accountable in all aspects of life, evil is satisfied. If we have no love, hope, or faith, evil wins.

There's a part of the story of my time on Mount Cutler that I haven't talked about, and that's the tears. I cried for a majority of that time on the rock. As the tears rolled down my face, I felt them hit my hands and finally found the missing part of the puzzle that I had been seeking. I already had love and faith, but I was seeking hope. I knew I had lost touch with everything. My vats were empty. I had so much love for the people in my life, I trusted God, but I was lacking hope. He saved my life that day and gave me hope. I know he can do the same for you.

CHAPTER 2
THE NEGATIVITY CLEANSE: A FOCUS ON MENTAL HEALTH

"We can complain because rose bushes have thorns, or rejoice because thorn bushes have roses."
— Abraham Lincoln

A strange metaphor for my journey from depression to hope came from my car. There is a VW (Volkswagen) emblem which is the handle to open the trunk of the car. It was an aftermarket carbon fiber piece I bought from eBay. After constant use it began to crack and peel. I started to notice it peeling more and more, and I felt a strong correlation with how I was digging deeper into the hidden layers of my own soul. I felt God speaking to me through a piece of plastic! As time went by I kept discovering things about myself that didn't seem to exist before. Each layer brought with it its own thrill, I never knew I could be so thoughtful and empathetic, I didn't know I had so much goodness and kindness within me. I remember someone cutting me off in traffic, and instead of chasing her down like I would have on a normal day and letting out a barrage of swear words, I simply smiled and thought that perhaps she was having a difficult day. It was such a pleasant change. I transformed from a completely confused, paltry, and hopeless human into a joyful and excited, real human, with hopes of making the kingdom a better place. This small little emblem was an incredible reminder of how we are so quick to forget or neglect the little things in life. We often skip over these important signs and go on ahead with our own plans. I believe we all need to be on constant notice and stay present as well as maintain a heightened state of consciousness. Having this awareness was one of the most influential inspirations that has ever happened to me. Every day I changed something small in order to grow and it ultimately made me into someone who wanted to serve. After seeing the repercussions from years of poor decisions, I knew that this time I must be intentional with my time on earth and be more thankful.

The layers kept peeling and peeling. God was making me more aware, bringing me a purpose in life, and lighting a fire in my heart at the same time. I began filling my time with more positive people and activities and feeling joyful much more often because of it. That VW emblem, as small and unnoticed as it was, motivated me to keep digging. As I was scratching off the last few flakes from that emblem, I started to smile. I knew I was taking notice. Micah Tyler sings, in his song "Different," the following words: "I don't wanna hear anymore, teach me to listen. I don't wanna see anymore, give me a vision." A powerful reminder to continue seeking knowledge and following the narrow but right path. All of us need to seek our VW emblem. What is something in your life that may seem unnoticed to many but is staring you right in the face? What's your VW emblem story?

Now let's shift our focus onto mental health. Factors that can affect mental health include: unemployment, bereavement of a loved one, trauma, neglect, isolation, loneliness, stress and money, drugs, sleeplessness, alcohol and physical health. Without proper coping mechanisms, we eat ourselves alive with negative self-talk. "I'll never get better," "I'm not good enough for anyone, that's why I'm always alone, "I really should just die already, I'm not serving any useful purpose being alive." These were some of the phrases I said to myself at my low times. I also had physical pain in my leg, felt neglected, thus I abused pain medication. This was a recipe for disaster.

Statistics show that about one out of every five adults struggle with some sort of mental illness. These illnesses include depression, bipolar disorder, post-traumatic stress disorder, schizophrenia, eating disorders, borderline personality disorder, as well as mental illnesses sustained from drug or alcohol abuse. Serious mental illnesses cost America nearly $200 billion a year in earnings. Over half of American adults with a mental illness do not seek or receive treatment. The mental health of our youth is worsening as well; school shootings are increasing, and suicide rates are going up faster than at any other time in history.

There certainly are some disturbing facts out there on suicide. Firearms use accounts for about 50% of suicides, and suicide is the tenth leading cause of death in the United States. According to 2016 statistics, nearly 45,000 people a year commit suicide. The connection between mental health issues and suicide is not as simple as it sounds. Anyone can have suicidal thoughts and inclinations. And the sad thing is that we're not even paying enough attention to these issues. Our society has misplaced its priorities, and we're focused on things that don't have value while ignoring the important bits. We keep arguing about bullying and gun laws and we ignore the most Important thing which is human life.

Little steps like changing how we talk to ourselves can go a long way towards making a tremendous change. Becoming aware of the driving force for your fear is very important. And remember, everyone has negative thoughts, but you don't have to believe them! What are some of the activities that help you cope with stress? Mental health is not as simple as fixing the brain—your heart needs to be healthy and so does your mind. There are a whole lot of things that contribute to a mentally healthy life. And it starts, most importantly, with self-talk and how you view yourself. If you tell yourself you are going to have a bad day, then you probably will.

Whether you realize it or not, you may be a negative person. If you find yourself complaining all the time about the weather, people, traffic, or anything out of your control, then you need to make some changes. Bad things happen to everyone, not just you. You have a choice about how you will react to any situation, so take a deep breath and think through your response. We can also continue to work on our positive mindset by realizing that these are just thoughts entering our heads. They don't have to crystallize into words from our mouth. When you view negative thoughts like this, it becomes easier to keep them in check and neutralize them before they adversely affect your life.

Society often says, "positive vibes only!" but in our personal lives, we realize that it is just not that simple. In order to grow as humans, we need to hear criticism with an open heart and mind. For example, I know that I am not a great writer. I know that I am not good at much, but I do believe in myself, and I certainly don't believe in the word impossible. However, beyond myself, there is a God who believes in me, and with Him anything is possible. I no longer allow myself to talk down to anyone, including myself. I accept the flaws of the people around, and I hope others can accept mine as well. This will be a never-ending process in life but establishing this thinking now will help me grow so I can help others grow, too.

Mental health can be affected in both good and bad ways. If we filter out successes and focus on our failures, then you create a negative thinking cloud in your brain. Do not get attached to being perfect or right 100% of the time. Do not allow yourself to think just in black and white; life isn't that simple. There's black, white, grey, and fifty shades of grey (pun intended). No one is perfect, and no one is always right or wrong. Don't begin to attach labels. Calling yourself a loser or other idiots is pointless.

If you feel embarrassed, that does not make you dumb. Making decisions when you are emotional is not ideal, so do not rush to call yourself or other people names. Just like judging a book by its cover, jumping to conclusions is not helpful thinking. There are many types of thinking that go right over our heads and seem less important. There are some types of people who take responsibility for problems that are not completely their fault; thus, letting someone else off the hook for their own mistake. Constantly blaming yourself is not healthy! Another unhelpful thinking style is basically the same as being dramatic or blowing things out of proportion, using phrases like "everything sucks," or "nothing ever goes my way." It's important to identify the particular negative phrase that you often use and consciously replace it with something more positive and uplifting.

Another aspect of mental health is taking responsibility. If you're going to stay stable emotionally, you need to stop blaming your parents or the government or the weather for the things that are happening in your life. When you focus on blaming others, you are enabling negativity in your brain. Your perspective on everyone outside of yourself or who agrees with you becomes evil. Essentially, you are fanning the flames of hate and anger and your mind becomes completely troubled. Would you not agree that our culture has normalized sickness? Rather than puttlng mental health at the forefront, we put more focus on oral hygiene. Re-read that sentence—does that not sound messed up? Rather than getting an annual checkup on our brains and our thoughts, decisions, etc., we go to a dentist to get our teeth checked because that is more important to our society. How do we not have more support groups or ways to get help for our mental issues? Everything is full circle when it comes to mental health. If your parents, friends, or family are enabling you and letting you off the hook for mistakes or failures, then as a society, we are failing you. Everyone needs help, everyone needs accountability, and there is no way you can go about life without a community to provide feedback and constructive criticism about your decisions.

Mental health can shape everything in life. It can form habits, it can impact your decisions, it can affect your happiness, and it can alter your thinking. Are you a thermostat or a thermometer? Thermometers are simply measuring devices, they only measure the temperature in the surroundings, they respond to what the environmental conditions dictate. This metaphor can be used in all different areas of life. In business, if the thermometer in the room is cold, everyone in the meeting seems lifeless. If it is hot in the room, then people start arguing and conflict arises. A thermostat, on the other hand, is proactive, it's used to set the temperature. A thermostat dictates what the temperature should be rather no matter what the environmental conditions are. When we, as well as others, react in thermostat mode, we create an environment of precise, consistent, and effective thinking. Whether or not it is cold or hot in the room, leaders can adjust the temperature and use conflict positively or pump up the room with some motivational talk. When we use this metaphor in our personal lives it can be extremely beneficial for mental health. We should refuse to be thermometers simply going along with the negativity around us. Instead, we should be like a thermostat, and control our responses. We can refuse to sink into despair alongside other negative people, and instead maintain an attitude of cheerfulness and enthusiasm. As a result, we use this mentality to positively impact others in our lives. We motivate them to be better and grow. We combat the hate and anger with a smile or a laugh. Do not allow others to influence you like a thermometer does; instead, train your brain over and over until it becomes a habit, thus you become the thermostat that sets the temperature. What temperature are you trying to set?

The truth is that having a mental illness is just as bad as any sickness. When our brains become completely overtaken by negativity we rarely find ways to look past the tunnel we have dug ourselves into. There needs to be a change in our society, and I believe it should start in the schools. If parents are not doing a successful job at home with their children, then we must find a new way to help anyone who is suffering. From childhood to early teenage years, most people avoid talking about issues with their parents or siblings. Even as adults we find it difficult to be vulnerable to others by displaying our true emotions. We avoid being vulnerable and learn to hide our sadness, weakness, and fears. In some cases, we bottle up anger and bitterness so as to avoid confrontations. While these negative emotions are not bad in themselves (because they provide feedback about the state of our mind), bottling them up can be really toxic. Repressed emotions often lead to serious mental issues later in life. This could be just a small portion of the problem but tackling it will go a long way in helping to drive back the mental illness epidemic being faced by society. If the schools can teach children about life's difficulties and how to properly handle their emotions, then maybe we could start a change.

As a society, we also tend to put the blame on a thing, saying it is the problem rather than the person or their mental health. We try to outsource the culpability and make the person behind the act seem like a victim of circumstances beyond their control. All of the shootings that are happening and people being murdered are because of guns rather than the human. Drugs and alcohol are the problem, not the person abusing them. The brain is the cause, and the result of all of this is suicide, murder, and death. It seems to be increasingly difficult to remain sane in an insane world.

How can we stop school shootings? As a society, we have failed by using social media and other news outlets to glorify the school shooters. We plaster their face all over different platforms, giving them exactly what they want. School shootings rarely ever happened in the past, but now they are abundant. Why don't we hear more about achievement stories? Or times when a shooting was stopped?

There is a gaping hole in how kids are raised today in comparison to the older days. There is a huge lack of discipline and accountability for actions, and a lack of mentors for kids. Our society needs to act and speak up when we see anything suspicious. Most importantly, listen and spend some time with your children. They are the future and they need help, now more than ever.

We also fail as a society at showing love. Some of the outcasts in the schools are constantly overlooked by their peers. Let's change and show them we are all brothers and sisters. One of my favorite lines from a song is, "When I look into the face of my enemy, I see my brother." Why is it so hard to have this philosophy towards everyone? We read over and over about these school shootings across the country, and friends and family come out after the fact to say they knew the shooter had mental problems. As discussed before, these mental issues are not being addressed, and they are getting worse. No matter what, we need people to speak up sooner, because it could potentially save a loved one's life. Most of the time the warning signs are there, we just overlook them or choose not to speak up. Stop the bullying, stop the hate speech and the aggressive behaviors, and please speak up when you think someone needs help. If we can't teach people about God in our schools, at least we can teach them about love. Hope will build a house, while faith and prayer will not allow it to be torn down.

Alternatively, there is an obvious answer to solve mental illness and that would be medication. For many, medication is actually necessary and can be quite beneficial. The idea here is to be open to the idea of medication and not to avoid it out of stubbornness, because this could be the difference between life and death, between happiness and depression. Many people who struggle with depression or some sort of mental illness typically have a chemical imbalance. Think of how dynamic our bodies are and how billions of different chemical reactions create our mood or perceptions towards life. Your loved ones and/or doctor should be involved in your care as well. Why would you not want to get better? Do you really want to die? Or would you consider fighting for your life?

We all have been through some sort of pain that literally crushed us. Whether it be a break up, a job loss, injury, or maybe the death of a loved one. The pain always becomes intense and direct, almost as if a fire has been set at your feet and slowly creeps up your body until you're engulfed in sadness. Many people decide to take the wrong approach to solving their sadness. They decide that drinking, drugs, or sex are the answer, and they avoid the real issues. Distractions are just what they are: distractions. Temporary releases from the true problem. It certainly isn't easy to just face the issues head on and fix it. For some, it takes time, it takes a good cry, or a loud yell in the shower.

The only truthful way to fix sadness is to choose happiness. At the end of the day, you have a choice to make. Ask yourself, do I want to continue to be sad or will I consider happiness? Happiness comes from within. You have the choice to look at every situation, thought, or action in a negative light, or you can choose to smile, take control of the situation, and see it as an opportunity to be happy.

When I spent my time talking to patients with mental illnesses, I was able to draw quite a comparison between their thoughts and feelings. I was also able to understand how important it is to have hope and faith as well. Many of these patients did not have much hope for a brighter future or better days. On the other hand, I was very excited for the future, but I was dwelling in the present. Our brains are incredible, and our thoughts and emotions shape the manner in which we proceed through life. Trying to explain mental illness to someone who does not have it can be very frustrating. If you can't put yourself in their shoes, then you just won't ever understand. To fight these mental illnesses, we must continue to shape our minds with positive people, thoughts, and actions. Expecting to change overnight by sleeping more and eating healthier or whatever it may be is just a start. You must create healthy habits and continue following them daily until they become routine. This can ultimately create the positive environment that will help fight the mental illness. Everyone has bad days, but when you let bad days become bad weeks or months and so on, then you must make changes immediately.

And remember, even with as much encouragement as friends or family can provide, this all comes down to you making the decision to get better. If you strive for better days, let today be the day you start anew. Don't wait for some vague period in the future before you begin to act to regain your happiness. I had a good friend talk to me about being in "the cave," that dark spot where you can't escape your own thoughts and feelings. She spent eight months there, reading over 80 books and learning about several different topics. She shared with me that no matter what happens in life, if you even let the negativity in and dwell on it, you will become that. Although it was a dark time, rather than sulking and giving up, she chose self-development over giving up, and it changed her life.

CASE STUDY

I wanted to help my community out by using the knowledge I had gained on healthy living. I knew that most people constantly make the wrong decision when it comes to their health, and I had the knowledge and power to help. My experiences had revealed so much to me about mental health and I felt a responsibility to show other people how to go about it. Every day I get the opportunity to talk to someone I have never met before and tell them about the importance of diet, being positive, smiling and laughing more, and just enjoying life moment by moment. Because I knew the struggle and how easy it is to just say, *I give up.*

I always ask the same three questions with the patients I interact with at the hospital every day. Does your health limit you from doing what you want in life? What kind of changes can you make today to live a healthier life? What can I do for you to help you live this life? Whether this was God putting it on my mind or it was my calling, I know that simple little initiatives like this can impact so many. Many times, when I ask patients these questions, I get a wide range of answers. Most—and I when I say most, I mean around 88%—say that their life is just fine, they enjoy coming to the hospital when they are sick. Whether or not I was getting truthful answers from these patients is another thing I wondered about. After months and months of asking these questions, and talking to 723 different patients, 636 of them said they were either just fine, didn't want any help, simply avoided asking for help, or felt uncomfortable answering.

I never really question why people come to the hospital for help. Primarily because the hospital is a glorified beauty/mechanic shop for the human. The nurses, doctors, and therapists come in and out of their room trying to find ways to help.Hospitals and other healthcare facilities we have nowadays are immaculate. They offer incredible treatments, wonderful doctors and nurses, and top end care. Why would someone want to stay out of the hospital when they get more attention than they do in the real world? Personally, I think people would be discouraged to go to the hospital if they found out the rooms had no windows, televisions, or free Wi-Fi. Not that I am suggesting this type of change, but you get the gist. A hospital today is essentially a hotel with people who treat you well and want to make you feel like a king or queen. With the comfort provided by hospitals, people have an incentive to not want to get better.

I may be primarily focusing on the norm in the USA, which, as many know, is not a very healthy country with a lower life expectancy than the likes of Italy, Switzerland, Australia, or Singapore. The common denominator is that mental and physical health needs to be addressed. Our minds are filled with misinformation. Our habits are determined at a young age by what our parents or social groups find to be normal. Popular surgeon, Ben Carson, talked about this in his book, Think Big. Young people learn how to dress, talk, and even behave from movies and Hollywood stars, they hardly do any thinking for themselves. Rather than taking the time to educate ourselves and learn different ways, we stick with comfort. As shown in our immaculate hospitals, fast food, and television watching on the couch, we love being comfortable. Being someone who strives to challenge others, it was time for me to address this comfort.

People want to be taken care of; our natural instinct as humans is to be loved and cherished by others. And this is exactly what most hospitals nowadays provide anyone who is sick. Most of these patients I am interacting with are in and out of the hospital several times in a year, and they wonder why they aren't getting any better. We call them our frequent flyers. It's these 12% I am interested in most. Hopefully one day I can make that 12 a 13%, or even higher. These 12 percenters give me in depth answers, they have questions, and they seem intrigued by this young white guy asking such deep questions. Then I see the face I am looking for, the *look into the sky moment,* I like to call it. They start to question whether or not they are living a life they are okay with, and they wonder how it got to this point—and what now?

When it comes to finding the root cause of problems in this world, we have to start somewhere. Just as habits are conceived based on learned rituals, we must seek the source of why the brain decides to choose an unhealthy life that leads people to the hospital. Of course, I cannot include many other medical issues that are not caused by poor eating, drugs, alcohol, and genetics in this statistic. Unfortunately, there are many healthy people out there who do end up having various medical conditions that require visits to the hospital. I am primarily focusing on the population that wonders why they got lung cancer when they smoked a pack of cigarettes every day for 30 years. Or the people who never exercised and became obese, thus causing their heart to start failing, and so on.

Let's focus on these 12 percenters again for a minute. Why did they decide to be vulnerable and open up to me? Why did they decide that they now wanted to try and fix their health? Why did they become curious after I asked those reflective questions? I believe it was the hope to get better and to change. Everyone wants to be healthy, live a life they dreamed of, and become something great. Whether or not you think it's too late, it never is. You can make changes today to become someone totally different tomorrow. It all starts with attitude and willingness to change. Throw your stubbornness out the window and be open. Now you know why the rearview mirror is so much smaller than the windshield in cars. Your future is ahead of you, and the path is way bigger than your past. Those 12%, they have me up all night writing and inspiring me to make changes in my life to better others. They ask questions like; how do I change? Why do I always feel so sick? Why am I not getting better? I take this opportunity to say a few simple words. Smile and laugh more, eat better, and speak up when you want help.

Many of us go through life without asking these questions to the people who can help or want to. I was one of them myself for a long time. This goes back to the proactive and reactive decisions. Being reactive can cause a lot of pain for the future. Being proactive can help steer you away from making poor decisions that may lead you into a downward spiral. Whether this person I was visiting in the hospital was 20 years old or 80, they still got the same message from me. I hoped to hear them being joyful about life, passionate about their job, or just overall happy to be alive. For the 12%, I want to tell you that my attention is on you. How can I and how can we as a society help change the future? The desire to reach these 12 percenters grows every day. I want to know more about why they want to change, what drives them, and how we can turn that 12% into a much larger percentage of people.

For me, making a small impact in a few hospitals and nursing homes throughout Indiana and Colorado could mean a momentous change to the world. Little drops of water, they say, make a mighty ocean. If a few other people in other places also decide to similarly put in the effort to reach people, then we might have the chance of making a real change. Whether or not this actually happens is not my priority. I believe I was brought here to inform these hospital frequent flyers that they can live happier and healthier lives by making just a few minor changes.

Everyone is seeking some sort of attention or validation to hear they are doing the right thing. We all want to feel that we have found the correct path in life. Why do you think suicide rates are increasing? I have worked in many intensive care units and dealt with patients who attempted suicide, and I have noticed a trend that is quite disturbing. They constantly speak of feeling inferior, inadequate, embarrassed, and depressed. Personally, having dealt with depression, I can relate first and foremost to the notion that our society puts way too much pressure on people to be something that they are not. Social media is a huge contributor to this problem. Everyone else puts up the best version of their lives for others to see. And when most people see this, they develop an inferiority complex. They view themselves in the light of others' achievements and feel they're not worth much. Instead of lifting each other up, we use our displays of wealth and good living to make them feel low. Why are we more focused on telling people they have a problem than on trying to help them fix it?

The selfish type tends to give up on others because it's inconvenient for them to help. The selfless know they have an opportunity to potentially turn around someone's life by doing the right thing, and they are excited by it. Here comes the kicker though: We need to find a solution. For me, there really isn't anything other than love, hope, and faith. Everyone needs these three. If you have love in your heart, then you find it easy to forgive and forget. You learn to care for others, and you tend to be happier in general.

If you have hope, then you see light even in the darkness. You know that life can be tough but you're an optimist; always believing good times are ahead. And with faith, you believe that God has you covered—no need to worry because you trust in the source from which all is forgiven. Just imagine if you have all three working together at once. Now that is a powerful combination!

CHAPTER 3

FAILURE IS SUCCESS IN PROGRESS

"I can accept failure, everyone fails at something.
But I can't accept not trying."
– Michael Jordan

The process of writing a book is not easy. I had all of these great ideas in my head but no real content. I started to write for hours and hours, it was a sort of catharsis. I was literally bleeding my mind of its contents through my fingers on the keyboard. When I wasn't writing, I was recording myself. There were times where I felt like a madman, I was so excited about this book I just couldn't stop. I simply wanted to let it all out. I wrote, recorded, and journaled every day for a year. There were plenty of bumps along the road. I began getting frustrated by the fact that I had spent over three months composing this book, and realizing that I was only 10% done. Then the possibility of failure dawned on me. It occurred to me that I could actually flop and end up publishing something that no one would buy or read. Or worse still, I could even end up not completing the book at all.

This was another point over which I pondered. I realized that for most of my life, I had been a stranger to failure, and this was one significant thing that had held me back. It was the root of most of my problems. I always sidestepped ventures where I felt I was likely to fail. I had spent most of my life in my comfort zone. Now, with this book, I had failure staring me right in the face, and my first impulse was to do what I always did- run, stop trying. But I wasn't that man again, that layer had peeled off just like the Volkswagen emblem. I knew that if I would turn my life around, I needed to look fear right in the face and call its bluff. There was no assurance that I would be able to write a good book or that anyone would find my story interesting, but I had to try. And with that realization, I shook off the lethargy I felt and continued writing. I believed in myself and chose to write the book anyway. It was my first step to redemption. And you know what? You can take that step too! Yours might not be writing a book. It may be building a business. It may be asking someone you love out. It may be reaching out to a friend with whom you've had a bitter altercation. Whatever it is, if you never try, you'll never know. And no, I'm not going to tell you that you won't fail. You may actually fail, but failure itself is not as bad as we often think. It's only a stepping stone and a learning opportunity.

When you bend like a branch in a hurricane and you break into two, then you'll be able to understand what I mean when I say there is no other direction than up, because I have been there. Just remember that people all over the world are praying for you and me, the broken, the defeated, the hopeless. So why not be hopeful? You probably will only have one, maybe two, chances in your life to fix your brokenness, so you better take that opportunity when it comes. What will become of you?

It took me almost 15 years to actually dig into life. I had the right intentions—I just made poor decisions along the way to discovering life. The beauty is not in a bottle or a drug or on a cell phone. It's out there, with people and experiences, sharing love and kindness to all no matter who they are. When we look back to reflect on our lives, will we be happy with making someone cry over an argument we started? Will we feel fulfilled knowing that we made someone feel miserable for a mistake they made? People will constantly disappoint us if we let them, or we could try to be better ourselves and react positively when faced with difficulties. We should all continue to strive to help one another, as there is no greater feeling than making a difference in someone's life. It may be hard to believe, but the obvious saying is that the truth hurts.

The following is a background story of the physical pain I have both experienced and created throughout the years. Also, I am a fitting example of what not to do when it comes to seeking medical attention.

When I was a young, reckless, crazy kid, I drove my bicycle into the neighbor's house around the age of eight. Around that same age, I was flung forward in a minivan, slammed the dashboard with my face, and then blacked out. A few years later, I went in to the doctor's office but all of the patient rooms were full, so the nurse decided to give me a shot while standing up. My mother looked at a poster of a monkey and said, hey look, it's you! As the needle went in my arm, I laughed at my mother's witty joke, fell, and hit a chair, out cold again. I rolled in a Jeep Cherokee several times to wake up to a dangling finger and a split open head. Concussion count is at three. In high school, I was working at a hardware store when a lady decided that her cell phone conversation was more important than the safety of a young man putting a propane tank in her trunk. She then proceeded to shut that trunk on my head, causing me to collapse in the parking lot.

I was always playing sports. As I got older, I decided to try out soccer for the first time. In one of our recreational games, I was running at full speed and got pushed from behind. My left collarbone was the only thing separating at the point of contact when I met the 230-pound goalie in a collision. Then I had surgery to repair the broken bone and proceeded with therapy for a few months. A few years passed and there were no injuries worth mentioning, surprisingly. I thought to myself, let's try this soccer thing out again. There was no way I was going to have another major injury, right? Well, in one game, I was dribbling the ball when out of nowhere I was bulldozed by someone. I can barely recollect what happened. I just knew that feeling of extreme pain as I laid on the ground. My right collarbone broke this time. Another surgery, some more therapy, and I was again as good as new.

As you can tell, I was a very stubborn person at this point in life. I simply never learned my lesson. After realizing it was time to give up on my soccer career, I switched back to basketball. As you may be thinking by now, why have I not just quit sports altogether? During a game with our church league, I was going up for a rebound and came down to a loud popping noise. I landed on someone's foot and my ankle rolled badly. Everyone in the gym heard it. I thought my right ankle was just sprained. It couldn't have been broken, right? I decided not to do the smart thing and see a doctor because I was going on a trip to California. I knew I would be doing some hiking through Yosemite National Park and obviously walking around other locations, and postponing that trip was not an option. I tried to man up as much as possible, but something was just wrong. I had an intense pain that did not feel right at all. My stubbornness again held me back from seeking the medical attention that could have saved me years of pain.

I remember leaning down in the grocery store to grab something out of the freezer when I couldn't stand back up. My ankle was completely locked. After it sort of popped itself back into place, I decided it was time. I finally got the x-ray and MRI to find out that I had ruptured the talus dome in my ankle, requiring surgery. The surgery went well but the rehab and therapy did not. I got back to a point where I could run again, but the scar tissue and nerve damage associated with the surgery caused me to need a second surgery. This next surgery was about a year and half after the first. It went very well, but the difference this time around was that my mind was no longer desiring rehab, or therapy. A couple months went by and I sat and wondered to myself, why is it not getting better? Why am I no longer motivated to push myself to get the results I want? Negative energy, negative feelings, negative environment. For the first time in my entire life, I felt dead inside. I had absolutely no desire to fix my problems. One major poor decision led to several destructive outcomes. And that is why it is extremely important to be proactive in all that you do in life to avoid major consequences. Still to this day I have issues with my ankle and I feel concerned for my future with all my concussions. But as we're reminded in this quote by Karl Marx, "The only antidote to mental suffering is physical pain," we must realize pain is temporary, and in most cases, it helps us grow, as long as we never give up.

We train and push our bodies to limits they sometimes just cannot stand. Becoming more in tune with how your body reacts to different activities, knowing when to rest it, when to seek medical advice, or when to nurture it, is all very important. I pushed and pushed with physical therapy, training, and weight lifting to finally feel healthy again after my injuries. The countless hours of pain in the gym pushing and knowing that eventually I would get the results I wanted were well worth it.

The first step to getting to where you want to be starts with you. Being able to get up out of bed and have your mind set on the sole purpose of getting better may start with your physical health, with a workout, or mental health, with meditation. Whatever it is you decide to do, be intentional with your plan to grow. I have to point out that anything that may seem beyond your scope of things that are easy to accomplish, will always be worth it in the end. Success often, if not always, lies outside of your comfort zone. People may tell you that what you are doing is ludicrous, but if it brings you joy and fulfillment then don't think twice. There is no reason to be ashamed of what works. Many people are so shut off to change they never get to truly experience living life to its fullest.

Failure also comes in many shapes and forms. Communication seems to be one of the biggest failures for everyone. Just think about how difficult it is to have a great conversation with someone who is either angry, stubborn, glued to their phone, or closed off. The key here is to find ways to turn arguments and conflict into constructive and positive outcomes. Training your mind to be open to innovative ideas rather than seeing them as negative can go a long way. There will be times of clashing heads with colleagues at work over a project or disagreeing with your spouse over which restaurant to dine at. Remember that choosing to be angry in any situation will negatively affect someone other than just you. When people choose to be content, selfless, and happy, the world is a better place.

Communication will always be an essential product of a healthy relationship that promotes growth. So, when you ask yourself, can I do more with less? The answer is yes, find ways to make it happen. In fact, there is something to consider here as well. Have you tried simplifying your life in order to be more efficient? We should always be reevaluating how we spend our time because it truly is the only thing we can never get back in this life. Rather than talking over and over about your plans to make changes, take action. Quitting certain habits, starting positive new ones, whatever they may be, should start immediately. Thinking and talking about change can become redundant pretty fast. You could sit on a couch, building castles In the air about the how nice your life would be without that habit. Yet, you could get off the couch and go do that exact same thing. If you want these changes to happen, stop reading this right now and start! Like a Nike advert says, "Just do it!"

The willingness to risk failure starts within ourselves. We must accept who we are, accept our flaws, be vulnerable to people, be raw, but also be vigilant to learn more and empower others to be stronger and better.

Failure is a great word; if you failed at something then you've learned a way that does not work. Failure is progression. The blessing is that now you have the opportunity to succeed by understanding what failure is. I'm an advocate for failure, because learning from mistakes is key to personal growth. Everyone seems to be satisfied with what looks good, but what looks good may not be what is good.

What you are willing to do today can change your life forever. Taking time to put in the hard work to obtain your goal can be extremely difficult at times, but as everyone knows, it's well worth the outcome. You then become immune to the pain of failure and your optimism grows with every new idea or venture. Everyone knows that whatever is hard or uncomfortable will always help you grow as a person.

Don't forget that the past is done, there's no looking back. Correct your mistakes and look towards the future. We all make the mistake of looking back at the past for too long, but this only stalls our progress and delays us. Remove the rear-view mirror and focus on the windshield. Life is too amazing for regrets!

If there was a way to avoid this regret, wouldn't you chase it? Take some time right now to visualize that dream life of yours and think about the hard work that will be essential to obtain it. Can you start right now? What is holding you back? Train your brain to never accept instant gratification because if you don't you will constantly be anxious and disappointed. This world is filled with dashed expectations and constant letdowns. Friends will abandon you, companies will fire you, your car will break down, and you may even break a bone or two. But you have to soldier on regardless.

And this is where the idea of balance is so important. Once you get your mind focused on being content and accepting life's difficulties, then nothing can disappoint you. Learn to love yourself. Learn to accept your flaws, and others too, but don't ever stop being positive. The devil is powerful, and one negative reaction or decision can lead to a lot of anger. This can lead to losing control of your own thoughts and feelings. Which then leads to poor decisions and terrible outcomes. Therefore, it is very important to love yourself and know yourself. Identify the situations and circumstances that tend to make you vulnerable to making wrong decisions. Take time to understand what puts you in bad or good moods. It may be an activity or spending time with a certain individual, our attitude can be affected by anything. Having this knowledge is unparalleled. Imagine if you had no idea the friend you spend most of your time with was trying to bring you down and cause you to become miserable. Imagine if the job you worked at was only making you happy because of the freedom or money it provided when deep down you knew it was not a good fit. It all circles back to dreams and obtaining your perfect life. Find a way to get to that point through hope and faith and constant dedication.

Following your own path often leads to disaster. We as humans do not take quality time to process our thoughts or consider our actions very well. We just dream big and follow our hearts. As many of you know, our hearts are guilty of falling in love with something that takes time to prosper. Wanting it and needing it are two totally different concepts.

You must understand the process; it takes time for your dreams to evolve into reality. And many a time, we fail at achieving these dreams, but it shouldn't ever stop us from trying to reach them. God's plan for us is perfect, put Him in control and trust His will.

MOISE BRUTUS STORY

How is it that we can believe in Santa for eight years, but we can only believe in ourselves for eight seconds? Comeback stories are inspirational, and they may even become the hope for our own comeback or recovery. God specializes in new beginnings and second chances. Although it is difficult to see beyond the present, we are often eager to see what the future holds. Will we ever recover from a heartbreak? A job loss? A health crisis? These and many other questions make our minds murky and hold us captive. What people need to hear is a relatable comeback story that can cause a chain effect and inspire them to change for the better. Using this book as a platform, I want people to be aware that this is my comeback story. I was messed up, I made very poor decisions throughout life, lied a lot, hurt many friends and was not the bright light I knew I needed to become. There was something burning inside of me that I knew needed help, but I was too weak to admit it to anyone. Thankfully God gave me my wakeup call on Mount Cutler in Colorado, so I could start my comeback story. I never intended to write a book for fame or money; I want to use this as a platform to tell others that change is possible, you can start loving more, and you can forgive 77 times seven like Jesus said.

Success does not come without belief. Change also does not come without belief. On an individual level, change occurs with persistency and dedication as well as belief. Rarely do individuals succeed on their own without a support group. When you are in a community or social group that believes they can make a change and encourages it as well, another small win occurs, and change happens. Encouragement plays such a vital role in change and growth. There are many days when the weather is bad, and it seems unfathomable to go exercise, but having a good friend hold you accountable can make a huge difference.

We only have so much willpower. It seems that eventually, when it wears down, we naturally fall into old habits. And when this breakdown occurs, we need to know there is not a lapse in growth. Developing positive habits such as reading, writing, drawing, painting, or just learning in general would be a great catalyst for a growth mindset. As in all of the previous habits or hobbies mentioned, it takes time to engrave them into your routine. We all know how easy it is to turn on Netflix rather than go for a walk. None of these practices are easy—personally, I struggle with this area in my life and my focus has been specifically on this. Knowing the triggers and being aware of them will help you when you start the change. My natural tendency is to turn on either the computer and play video games or get in front of the television and watch sports. Acknowledging that neither of these activities ever provided growth, I had to identify new ways to stop the routine. If we are being honest, rarely do this binge watching, screen staring times on the couch provide personal growth. Of course, even recreation has its place when done in moderation, but it's important that we are aware of it. Most people are drowning in over-indulgence and indiscipline without even knowing it.

Competition can be great, but more often than not, it creates division and conflict. Winning becomes the only thing that matters in sports. Rather than using competition as a chance to help others grow and become stronger, we constantly strive to win. This mentality does not last, and the euphoria of winning is fleeting. After witnessing several CrossFit competitions over the years, the overall conclusion is that this community creates a powerful and positive competitive environment. These athletes are constantly encouraging others to be better, stronger, and faster through motivation. Now, if we could only use this mentality in all aspects of life, then we could grow and be more united. Losing provides room for growth, and it also should become the motivator to work harder and be better next time. We need to continue to work on creating growth through competition rather than division.

I truly am inspired by brokenness. You will constantly see people who overcame harrowing, excruciating, and even tormenting situations to become prodigious stars in the world. The odds look overwhelming, but so are the stories of people who beat them. Why can't you be the next?

The next comeback story is one of the most influential stories I have ever heard.

It will always serve as encouragement for me to never stop growing and never ever stop believing in myself no matter the circumstances.

His name was Moise Brutus. He was a student at Miami-Dade College in Miami, Florida. At the time, Moise was only 20. He was riding his motorcycle on the Florida Turnpike in Miami on a nice October day in 2010. Out of nowhere, something crushed him, flying through the air and landing in a ditch near the road. Unfortunately, whoever ended up hitting him didn't stick around to help. Brutus was conscious but was bleeding very badly. He tried to reach for his cell phone with his left arm, but there was nothing there below the elbow. His legs were both gone too. Just imagine the shock and thoughts that would race through your mind if this happened to you. Mo, as he liked to be called, was fortunate enough to have one remaining limb, his right arm, so he eventually managed to get his phone and dial 911. An officer named Carlos Villalona responded to the call and said that Brutus's injuries were similar to wartime damage. Villalona had previously served in the U.S. Army. These injuries were certainly not common to see on someone who was still breathing. Brutus woke up three days later from a coma. He looked down and simply couldn't believe the sight. First thing he said was, "Oh my god, my life is over." For the next six months or so Moise just sat in a dark room and never left. He calls these the dark days for a reason. At his lowest point he weighed only 76 pounds. His mother was extremely worried and close to losing hope completely. They were on Medicaid, and getting help was certainly not easy. Mo knew he had two options: Stay in a clinical depression for the rest of his life or fight and become something incredible.

He once mentioned something powerful that really put life into perspective for me. He said that it was amazing to think life for him started after losing three limbs, and that it got even better. He started to appreciate every day of being alive and wanted to celebrate it. Brutus is a triple amputee. Mo's recovery had stalled under the old Medicaid. Thankfully, there was a private Medicaid insurer called WellCare that would start him on the path to recovery. His mother previously had to change his bandages and constantly run him to the emergency room when he was with the old Medicaid insurer. Mo said he was overly medicated during this horrible time too. WellCare changed his life forever. He was able to get incredible care, some of the best prosthetics in the world—basically everything he would ever need to turn around his life. Medicaid reform in Florida gave Mo some options that were not offered previously. The old Medicaid system prolonged the pain and suffering he had to endure before he was able to get life-changing help. In other words, WellCare's privately managed insurance, which is patient-centered, motivated Mo to get better. WellCare had a reputation to build, they had competitors in the market to beat, and this drove them to provide top notch care. Once again, let's look back on what I previously mentioned about competition and compare it to Mo's situation. A private company was able to help turn around someone's life just by offering a service that our government could not help with. This is a great example of how competition in the healthcare business ended up being the saving grace for Moise.

This traumatic experience led to something even greater for Mo as well. Although doctors said he only had about a 1% chance of survival after the crash, he knew that this could not be what would define him for the rest of his life. He ended up joining amputee support groups and slowly his attitude and outlook on life began to change. He got a dog named Dexter, whom he would walk around the block every afternoon. Dexter became his best friend. And then he did outpatient therapy to venture out of his comfort zone even further. One day during therapy, his therapist put him on a stationary bike. He never looked back. He now works out five times a week, cycles around 100 miles a week, goes to school, and is totally independent. Mo says when he is on his bike he feels free like the wind, and his disability doesn't even cross his mind. The small mention from a physical therapist gave Moise a newfound passion and belief in himself.

Mo began training for the 2016 Paralympics in Rio de Janeiro with the goal of representing the United States. One of the most renowned colleges in the world for cycling, Marian University in Indianapolis, Indiana, saw Brutus's ability. Making this particular team was not easy. They were made up of some of the best cyclists in the world. Marian's program has won 27 team national championships in track, road, BMX, and cyclocross. Brutus became the first amputee to join the team since Marian's program was founded back in 1992. Cycling was a perfect match for him. He thinks his story is simple and states, "I think my story is just one of not giving up."

Brutus wants to use his story to inspire others on their own journey. He uses his drive, compassion, and focus on doing this for unselfish reasons. Talk about a story of perseverance! From his motorcycle crash to becoming a collegiate athlete, he has quite a remarkable story. Brutus never wants people to start thinking about his missing limbs, but rather about overcoming any adversity that may end up coming along the road of life. Brutus continues to be a motivation for his teammates when they don't feel like practicing or feel tired. He is the ultimate encouragement to keep going and push harder. Teammates constantly say that he has the biggest drive and the strongest heart on the team. "Bad stuff will happen. You've just got to continue and not give up," said Brutus.

His story, like many out there, reminds me that hope is an essential component for growth. I have always felt like it was hard for me to trust people who are unbroken. But rather than thinking that way, the best philosophy is to teach people the idea that adversity and low times will always provide a chance for growth. And when you are in this moment, and the people around you keep saying it will get better, remember that the past is the past. It is hard to see through the dark days, but just like Moise Brutus, I can definitively say that is the truth. Better days are ahead, and you will have a newfound appreciation for life. You just have to believe. I was fortunate enough to get in contact with Mo on LinkedIn and we chatted a bit. He spoke of the journey having some difficult struggles, but just like myself, he is a firm believer in hardships building character.

He left with me a simple but powerful phrase: Never give up!

CHAPTER 4
TURNING YOUR MESS INTO BALANCE

"Next to love, balance is the most important thing"
–John Wooden

During the dark days, I never had a feeling of inflicting pain on others; it was specifically toward myself. And in a way that contributed to my inability to get help quickly. I felt I wasn't hurting anyone, just myself, so there was nothing to worry about. But it was during this period I started to realize that even harming myself would in turn harm many others. My life was beyond just me alone. One of the many lessons God taught me right then and there was that it was time to start over. God was about to turn my mess into my message. If we sit down and think about it, how amazing is life? To be able to take a breath is in itself perfect.

So while we all are here, let's stop creating labels and categorizing people, bullying and ostracizing others. Let us all see that we can change someone's life with small and simple actions, and hopefully create a better world from it.

Have you ever felt terrified to tell someone you need help? Are there issues you constantly avoid talking about with your loved ones? Vulnerability is tough, and we have so many masks we wear in this life: self-loathing, elated, animosity, joyous, melancholy, thankful, pessimistic, caring, and sometimes just pure evil. We are afraid that exposing our real selves will make people avoid us, judge us, look down on us or even hate us completely. Well it's true. A lot of people will be uncomfortable with the real you after the mask falls off. But you know what? It's the beginning of change. While some people will leave, others will appreciate your honesty. When you take these masks off and show your true self, you connect on a much deeper level with the people in your life. And you can only begin to get better when you allow your true self to be revealed. We all want to be better people, so why not be open to the idea of making changes? If you want to be a better friend or partner by admitting you are pessimistic, then they should be aware and thankful you are making the effort to work on this. If they are not, do not be discouraged; continue to work on being that positive light. We tend to shut down when we hear something that upsets us. We reject it in our minds and let it take control. I say, be vulnerable, have an open mind, speak from the heart, and find ways to improve yourself for the benefit of others. You must be willing to commit to deep change within yourself. Becoming aware of old patterns that cause regression and finding ways to alter them. Focusing on loving above everything. We are nothing without love.

How can we create this balance from our mess? Let's discuss some examples we all experience in life.

Restless Nights: Rolling back and forth in bed with our minds going full speed. Disturbing dreams or even nightmares. That feeling of comfort that your sheets provide, or maybe the soreness of your body, makes you want to never get up. Rather than being frustrated with whatever is causing this pain, what if we just lie still? We could allow our mind and body to connect without even moving or opening an eyelid. If we can take this posture and remain relaxed, our bodies will begin to release tension and ease our minds. This sort of practice is very important in prayer and meditation.

When we allow our heart to be open and focus on our breathing, the mind tends to clear, and the stress and anxiety begin to wither away.

Negative Self-talk: Sometimes, we talk ourselves into justifying the negativity in our lives, "I'm not the only one; I'm not the only one to neglect a relationship. I'm not the only one to get addicted to pain medications. I'm not the only one to disrespect my family. I'm not the only one to lie to my loved ones. I'm not the only one who feels lost in this world. I'm not the only one who wants to end it." When I went back and thought of these individual statements, I felt saddened. I knew that this old self needed to disappear. There was no longer time or space to live in that world. There is a bright future ahead and sulking in this negativity was not going to help me grow. Whether it is insecurities, doubts, or fear crippling us inside, we have to become aware of it, and then fight it. The longer we let these thoughts control us, the more they eventually become us. If you are able to identify them, then you have a head start on some people. I let this negativity consume me for years and was oblivious to the pain it was causing in my life.

Regret: It's such a nasty word that should never even be in your vocabulary. If you have regrets, it means you did not take time to analyze the outcome before making a decision or decisions. You can't expect any poorly thought through decision to have a positive outcome. See the big picture, stop doing the second-guessing game. Process your decisions before they become actions. It is much easier to do the right thing the first time around, but if you don't, remember to ask for forgiveness when you have lied, and be honest. The main mistake I made in my past was not truly analyzing my thoughts and actions, I just went with what felt right in my gut, which felt good going down, but when regurgitated, tasted similar to a sickness. The foundation for successful relationships is trust and forgiveness. Learning from your mistakes can be quite challenging, but forgiveness comes from God. He believes in you above anyone else.

Balance does not come from material things.

Solomon was said to be the wisest king to ever rule Israel. In Ecclesiastes he experimented with excess and it left him feeling the same desire for what our hearts eternally long for, God. Ecclesiastes 1:2 says, "Meaningless! Meaningless!" says the Teacher. "Utterly meaningless! Everything is meaningless." Ecclesiastes 1:14: "I have seen all the things that are done under the sun; all of them are meaningless, a chasing after the wind." No activity or substance will ever fill the void you experience over and over throughout every day. Instagram, gin & tonics, marijuana, *Game of Thrones,* and even carrot cake won't fill that void. Find your balance. And remember that extremism in anything is not a healthy habit.

A balance between life and technology. It seems as if the smartphone controls our lives now. We rely on it to wake us up in the morning, to give us news, to catch up on trends, to communicate, to pay bills, to shop, to read, and the list goes on and on. When did this happen, and why? When has a smartphone ever truly brought you pure joy? I have noticed that life is amazing without devices. Less TV, fewer video games, and less social media, time texting, and reviewing restaurants means more time being, doing, and living in the now. Picking up a book or a cup of coffee and having a conversation with a friend is more meaningful than hash-tagging your latest piece of pizza. Developing strong relationships will never happen over a text message or a phone call; we need face-to-face communication. We need nonverbal communication, smiles, laughter, and real emotions to capture this amazing feeling of love and connection. Phones should never be more valuable than human connection.

We must also stop the focus on problems in this world or our lives and shift them onto solutions. Just for a while, turn off anything that beeps, rings, or buzzes—thus eliminating all distractions. Understand that life is 10% what happens to you and 90% how you react. You will always have a choice in any situation. Be more intentional and make plans before you start something. Another helpful idea to remove some stress is by keeping a note pad or booklet near your bed. Many of us awake throughout the night for various reasons; if your brain can't shut off, start to jot down what you are thinking. Review this in the morning and learn from it. Hopefully over time you will notice a better-rounded, more positive mindset through your writing.

Because our minds tend to drift too often. It is said that your typical smartphone owner looks at their phone over 2600 times in a day. Sadly, I would say at times in my life I was a part of this statistic. Now I realize some people need their phone for work and that is understandable but remember that it should only be for work and not pleasure. Most people have way too much dependence on their phones. The amount of time you can instead spend conversing with friends, family, or doing any physical activity will be of great benefit for your mental health. Productivity is a key foundation for happiness or fulfillment. It may seem like work at first but reaching the finish line with anything gives the mind a sense of achievement, thus building our self-confidence.

There really is nothing impossible for you to achieve. As mentioned several times throughout this book, you must have self-control. This all starts with practice, teaching the brain when and when not to act upon our thinking. Acting on every impulse is typically not a smart decision. The lifestyle of being clean of negativity and thoroughly focused on a positive all-round approach takes time and is not easily attainable. We all struggle with urges for more of this or some of that which, deep down, we know is probably not a positive decision. As previously mentioned, focusing on small daily habits first and building on that will shape you into a powerful role model.

Working hard, eating healthy, giving gifts, contentment, and being slow to anger are the attributes I am constantly seeking for myself. I overemphasize how important it is to have a positive mindset at all times. It will constantly fight for you and combat all of the negative thoughts that enter your brain. So as you begin working on yourself and learning which steps to take to live a better life, remember that this process takes hard work and dedication. This is where you have all the power to make a difference for the rest of your life. Shape your mind around hope, faith, and love, and block all the negativity that even tries to enter.

I had to deal with a serious amount of neglect over the past few years, in all aspects of life, spiritual, emotional, physical, and mental. Quickly I found out that my world can crumble without balance. What do you think of when you hear the word neglect? I neglected a friendship I dearly miss? I neglected my spiritual life? I neglected my partner? I neglected my own self and what I love? This is why it is extremely significant to reevaluate where you are heading in life on a weekly if not daily basis. Reflecting and analyzing on everyday thoughts and decisions will fine-tune the brain. There are way too many distractions in the world, from television to social media, all dead and wasted energy. When taking the time to understand why it is you do what you do, your awareness for making smarter decisions comes more naturally. Balance is so important in life, and when neglect takes over, trouble is ahead. When you are not present, and you just run through the routine of everyday life, you lose touch with growth. You become stagnant and wasteful of the incredible talent and beauty that God created in you.

Neglect can be difficult to see when you are constantly focused on life and work, your normal routine has been neglected but you probably don't currently have the vision to see that. I constantly talk about developing healthy habits, making the right decisions and keeping balance, because then neglect rarely happens.

Most people instinctively think of the balance between work and life, but if you are working joyfully, then there is nothing to worry about. You can have a job that you look forward to and then life will fall right into place. A key to balance is also taking time away from the normal every day or week routine. Traveling, taking long weekends away from your city, vacationing, or serving on a mission trip can refresh the soul.

You can create more freedom in your life by being proactive too. A sloth won't accomplish anything, but haste leads to waste as well. Work smarter and more efficiently than your peers. Psalm 128:2 says, "You will eat the fruit of your labor; blessings and prosperity will be yours." Balance is always an ongoing process. If you continue to practice finding balance, then eventually you will find it.

Unfortunately, the world and our society put us under intense pressure to be busy. And because of this, we rarely find the time to reflect on our decisions. We constantly express our feelings through photographs, tweets, posts, and quotes, and often we don't analyze the impact it may have on others. We get attached to the idea that likes on social media equals popularity and approval.

And many of us think we need to work harder and longer hours despite feeling overworked and burnt out. Just like everything previously stated in this book, we need to continue to seek answers by being open and asking others for help. Rarely do people who feel frustrated or overburdened become motivated to work harder. The stress overcomes them and then they start to slip, give up, and even fail. Remember how important balance is and find ways to get it. You are not alone if you are feeling stressed or overworked; nearly 25% of the workforce feels the same way. A question to ask yourself is this: Are you really too busy to focus? Or, do you think you are too busy when in reality it's not busyness but rather being preoccupied?

There were also times in my life where I was consumed by work. Other times it was video games, sports, traveling, and so on. I got stuck in this pattern for so long that I was trapped in a one-track mindset. I had lost the balance that is so important to stay level-headed. Moderation needs to be understood, because being extremely involved in something makes you neglect other areas of life. Think of a time when you had little balance in life. What were the causes for this? How did you fix it or overcome the imbalance? This brings me back to talking about creating lists and being more organized. Understanding how you spend your time and when you are most effective is key to a balanced life.

Most people can relate to a time when they wanted to give up. Whether it was quitting a job or school, or maybe ending a relationship. These are the trials and tribulations that everyone has to face in life. No matter how hard it is, we should all learn to take a risk or to adapt, enjoy the struggle and fight through the pain. When I reflect back on my life, I had to quit playing sports after multiple injuries and it took several years to find other hobbies I was passionate about. This is where being well rounded can be such a tremendous asset to people who face adversity. Because once you get to the point where you no longer can do what you love, you end up being forced into change.

I was not prepared to give up on playing sports. I had done sports all my life but giving it up was what I ended up needing to do. I started to discover I had a strong interest in reading and writing. And as these interests grew, I enjoyed more conversations, I opened up a new part of my brain that wanted to learn more. Whatever happens in our lives, we must learn to be proactive when adversity comes our way. And remember that you are not the only one who struggles. If people were honest they all would say they struggle with something every single day. Becoming aware of how your brain thinks and how you react can help shape your life into an unbelievable moment to moment experience. For me, I became accustomed to having life pretty easy, somewhat handed to me on a platter of gold, and I noticed that my humility deteriorated when I was able to get what I wanted all the time. Being a home owner, working from home, coming and going whenever I wanted and living in amazing cities. Even reading that sentence makes me sound like a jerk. I was living the American dream, yet I was less thankful than ever. I was out of tune with the world around me, and once I had my meltdown it was way too late. Once again, this all comes full circle to finding balance, being content, and accepting your lot in life.

CHAPTER 5
HEALTHY HABITS

"We are what we repeatedly do. Excellence, then,
is not an act, but a habit."
– Aristotle

How can we be better for others? Listen. Stop judging or arguing and simply listen. Whether or not you have differences with others is irrelevant. Being respected and heard is what we want. We want that unconditional love that we get from our God to come from people as well. Many of my close friends in life are on opposite ends of the spectrum when it comes to various topics, but this has and never will change my opinion of them. We need to instill this thinking of love for all people regardless of who they are or what they believe. I believe that less violence and hate would happen if we began shifting our thinking toward others rather than on our own pain.

Start with being thankful for any little thing you can think of. Continue to press on no matter the pain, and always remember that it could be worse. Some people skate by in life without many consequences, a silver spoon handed to them when they were young, and money to help them get what they want and where they want to be in life. And others were dealt tough hands like family health issues, abusive parents, poverty or drug use, and for them, times were much tougher. I believe we all should face some trials and tribulations that push us to the brink. If you can't deal with pain, then you will never grow. Learning to cope with loss and struggle will always make you stronger. The feelings can make you numb at times, but remember to reflect upon the good memories and smile. Embrace the suck, soak it all in, and come out on top.

Healthy habits come with change or adaptation. Successful companies have a foundation centered on this idea. Create a positive environment, teach the employee how to successfully do their job, and everything else comes naturally based on new habits formed. The idea is centered on a growth mindset rather than being static. Most of us would all agree that we are set in stone on many different topics in our lives. This willingness to change or be open to new ways is the type of mindset we should all develop. As we talked about before, our natural tendency is to be selfish. This selfishness tends to rub off somewhere in our busy lives. Maybe this selfishness causes problems at work, in a relationship with your spouse, or in your relationship with God. Wouldn't it be nice to just have balance in life with no anxiety?

This society tends to give up too easily; when stress or problems arise, we run away. And everyone deep down knows you just can't run away from your problems. They will follow you to the next city, relationship, or job. If as a society, we decide not to address issues, whatever they may be, then we simply cannot grow. Leaving important issues unaddressed will prevent others from being able to help or save us. I have personally been at fault concerning this plenty of times. Now that I have the awareness, I can continue to work on it, and push others as well. There are so many benefits to conflict that most people do not realize. Having a willingness to listen shows respect. Whether you agree or disagree with this person is irrelevant, because everyone deserves a voice and respect. Put your opinions and politics aside for a second and just listen.

I'm a firm believer in lists, as you can tell. There is no one better than yourself for accountability. Your lists should consist of strict goals, plans, ideas, or statements that require attention. I'm not talking about something simple like a grocery list; instead, these should help you live a more organized and productive life. As stated before, our minds are so clouded we rarely remember to get important tasks done. If you are trying to work towards a goal, then making some sort of list is essential. Whether you want to graduate college, become a doctor, move to a different country, be a missionary, or lose some weight, having a list for it can be very helpful. These can be motivators to show progress as well. Rarely do people continue pushing through difficult life goals when they do not vividly see progress. I have been on the failing end of life goals more often than not, but now it is engrained in my mind to keep trying and never give up. Focus on small wins, for they become incentives and create a positive movement. Spread this among your friends, family, or coworkers, and you create an environment for success. When others pick up on this and run with it as well, then you have created a tiny culture around the idea of change.

Now that we have found our balance, let's find a way to challenge this existence by trying something outside our comfort zone. Some examples may be rescuing a dog, giving a stranger a hug, paying it forward at Starbucks, or donating your time to benefit someone other than yourself. Find someone or something to fight for. I was broke, depressed, and hopeless. I needed to take action. My story of being on Mount Cutler was the turning point in my life. Everything at that point had become clear: I wanted and needed to fight for a better life with or without whoever wanted to come along. I was choosing honesty, happiness, and selflessness as my path. My dream to become an accomplished writer, a C-level employee, a disciple, and a public speaker all gave me a true sense of passion and hope. I started writing because I had so much to share about personal failures that I knew I could connect with the sad, angry, and hopeless types. There is no greater satisfaction in life then turning someone else's story around for the better. Many of my friends and family chose to be that shining light for me, and to them I owe it all.

Whether this is on your brain or not, take some time to answer the following questions with complete honesty. Are you anxious or scared about anything in your life? If so, why? What can you do to overcome this fear or anxiety? Fear tends to control our decisions and actions much more than you'd think. This fear is so powerful, it causes some of us to essentially kill ourselves trying to be perfect. That fear of failure or rejection and even criticism holds us captive. Fear can even cause us to say yes when we mean no, and no when we mean yes. Fear is so powerful that it causes inner pain and, in worst case scenarios, depression or hopelessness.

We numb this fear with drugs, alcohol, sex, TV, or even excessive busyness. How do we get to the point where we realize these are just temporary band-aids, which in turn cause even worse inner pain? My demons held me in this state of hopelessness for way too long. As stated before, I was so hopeless I was one slip, jump, fall, or even negative thought away from ending my life. If we are able to identify our inner demons, why do we avoid fixing them? And why do we mask these demons with lies? We are lying to ourselves!

When fear is controlling us, just ask why. Question this fearful thought; try to find out if there is any validity to the fear itself. Many of our fears are not just created in our minds, they are external, forced on us by the media and people around us saying how awful the world is. If you really believe the Universe is out to get you, then you will struggle with trust and your anxiety and fear will get worse. The biggest help for this sort of pain can be fixed with something as simple as meditation. When you take time to reflect on what you are thankful for, a sort of awakening begins. Take some much-needed time for solitude and quiet time. The intentions of these sorts of reflections are to create new, healthy habits and to reshape our minds with those healthy habits.

Rather than being so negative saying "I can't, I won't, I don't know how", alter your thinking and start saying, "I will give that a try, I would love to learn, I think that would be a great idea!" The crazy thing about this type of thinking is that you literally have to train your brain on how to react to certain questions, situations, and experiences in life. This typically does not come naturally to humans. I was terrible at being positive towards trying new activities. I felt out of my comfort zone, confused, as if they were too difficult and not normal! Little did I know I loved most of these experiences; I had just preemptively decided they were not going to make me happy, which had already determined the outcome of fear, anger, frustration, or sadness. Part of this is due to the fact that most people are just too stubborn to try anything outside of their normal routine. If you think about it, why would you want to be completely shut off to new concepts or adventures? Try different types of food, riding a bike, or even traveling to a new city with the sole intention of creating new experiences.

Once again, remind yourself of this: Yesterday is gone, forget your bad memories, be optimistic about the future, and always have faith. This attitude is key for everything you do. I have lived in the past, I have sulked over memories, and I have seen doubt in my future and questioned my faith. All of this came from my inner negativity. That is why I am constantly reminding myself and others that you must surround yourself with positive influences, or at least be able to block out the bad. And always love, for hate will get you every time.

This all comes back to training your brain on how to react in certain situations. Rather than putting yourself at risk for consequences, think about taking the high road and setting yourself up for success. It may not be the most fun thing to do but doing what is right should always be the higher priority. It is so easy to fall into a trap of poor decisions; they become second nature. Everyone knows what their core issues are, or someone probably has made you aware of them at least. Why is it so difficult for us to address them and make changes? Is it stubbornness, pride, selfishness, or arrogance? I have to believe that we all simply don't want to change because of these reasons. Once again, I challenge you to take a major step in one area and make a positive change for someone in your life. It could be as simple as taking a friend to work out with you, or to church. Maybe it is helping your grandparents mow their lawn or driving a friend to the airport. Start with doing something out of your norm and watch what impact it makes. I can guarantee that you and whoever you helped will be grateful.

I am the first to admit that my stubbornness and pride kept me from trying out healthy habits that literally saved my life later on, meditation being one of them. Just like anything in life that can be beneficial or help us grow, meditation deserves a try. If you find yourself distracted or losing focus, then you can take a different route to fix that problem. It takes time and practice to become better and see results. Please do not be quick to judge without using your own personal experience as a baseline for your reasoning. Our minds are constantly flooded with thoughts and questions, so learning to take some quiet time and see results takes hard work and discipline. For me, I want to strive towards becoming as excited as Mark was in the Bible to tell the gospel to everyone with so much enthusiasm, yet also feel unhurried with my walk with Jesus.

This high-speed world we get caught up in does not seem to allow for silent time or meditation. Rather than taking five minutes, just 300 seconds, to sit in silence and think, we grab the smartphone or turn on Netflix and let the distractions engulf our lives. Many statistics show that humans touch, type, swipe, or click our phones over 2,000 times a day and spend an average of over 140 minutes using them. What did we do before cell phones? I remember the only problem I had when I was a child was when the basketball rolled under the car parked on the street and got stuck underneath.

We need to continue to seek the awareness of what controls our lives and find out why we become so anxious and fearful because of it. This pain that comes from fear can be overcome, and we can use it as fuel for change and growth, both as individuals and as a society. This type of thinking shifts our mindsets towards selflessness, participation and progress. On the other hand, if you live in fear, and anticipate that other people always want to hurt you, you become bitter, suspicious and defensive. Just because someone has wronged you does not mean that everyone has this intention. Whether it was a toxic relationship, a boss, or community you were part of, it does not mean that every relationship that ended poorly will happen again in the future. You must have this mindset and wisdom to know that the Universe has a difficult but sometimes also funny way of working things out for the better. Many, like myself, find this to be so difficult when our minds aren't right. Once you release your fear and anxiety, hope and strength come. We begin to see the light at the end of the tunnel and start heading upward over the mountain.

There will be moments where you think everything is going swimmingly and life is amazing—write down everything going on in your life at those times and make sure they are positive or healthy. Many times, you will notice that you are completely unbalanced in one or more areas and changes must be made.

Remember that it takes 21 days to create a habit. Three full weeks of complete focus. Not the easiest thing in the world, but anyone can do it. Most people are embarrassed to admit they have pains, struggles, or issues. Welcome to life! Everyone, not just you, has these problems. One of the toughest tasks in life is admitting that these flaws are real and expressing them to people in your circle. We want to mask our problems with fake happiness and it ends up eating us alive.

POPE JOHN PAUL II'S STORY

Imagine this: 10,000 people in St. Peter's Square, Pope John Paul II visiting with an enthusiastic crowd of supporters in the Vatican City. They had all gathered to receive the blessing from the Pope. He was reaching out to shake hands, pray, and smile with each passerby. He turned to cuddle an eighteen-month-old child, and out of nowhere, a Turkish extremist Mehmet Ali Ağca took out his Browning Hi-Power 9mm pistol and unloaded multiple shots, striking the Pope in the Popemobile on May 13, 1981. The Pope was responsive as his secretary asked him, "Where?" The Pope responded with, "The stomach." "Does it hurt?" "Yes, it hurts. It hurts."

Many stories have been told about how the Pope himself had blessed a new ambulance the day before by saying, "I also give my blessings to this ambulance's first patient." This ambulance would be the one that picked him up. Ironic? Pope John Paul II was in bad condition. After he was rushed to the hospital, doctors performed surgery for nearly four hours and had to remove multiple parts of his intestines. Just a few hours after the shooting, the Vatican was filled with mourners who had no idea whether or not he would survive. Many were seen praying and also in shock over what transpired. This same Turkish extremist had threatened to kill the Pope just two years before this incident. Pope John Paul II would miraculously survive the attempted murder and recover in the hospital while the assassin would be sentenced to life.

The beauty of this story came after the recovery and sentencing. The Pope spent time visiting Ağca in prison and continually asked people to pray for him whom he had sincerely forgiven. John Paul II said, "What we talked about will have to remain a secret between him and me. I spoke to him as a brother whom I have pardoned and who has my complete trust." His Holiness actually intervened to help secure Ağca's release from prison in 2000. Later, after Ağca had been released from prison, he visited the tomb of John Paul II and laid flowers at his grave. A truly remarkable story of forgiveness, selflessness, and hope.

It's pretty simple: Selfless people give, while selfish people make life complicated for others. Ask yourself these two questions and take some time to reflect on the answers. Do you gravitate towards helping others before yourself? Or, do you feel as if this is your world, and who are all these people trying to occupy it? You should seek out the selfless. The Jesus, Gandhi, Martin Luther King Jr., or Mother Teresa types. They will provide peace and show how grace brings beauty and happiness into life. The selfish types tend to be unpredictable, lacking humility, constantly manipulating situations, and lacking real empathy. The selfless types forgive and forget, volunteer their time and skills, empower others, and congratulate others on their successes. Constantly being consumed with your own problems will drain the energy needed to act selflessly. Pay attention to what is going on around you and in the world; it should provide some perspective. You are just a speck of sand in this endless universe, but knowing this is one thing, understanding it and living in its consciousness is another.

Here are some ideas to help you become more selfless. Find a workplace that makes you happy yet also provides a service for others. Donating your time or money without expecting a reward is good practice as well. Stop thinking of ways to avoid giving; instead, train your brain to be the helper. Surround yourself with people who are selfless, and you may learn a thing or two. We all know it's much easier to just be selfish. Plain and simple. If you finally lose control and no longer have people giving you the love that you desire, your selfishness will leave you feeling angry and alone.

Reflect on situations that are typical daily encounters. That stranger you just walked by could have just lost their job or a loved one, so smile and say hello. Don't just open a door for a lady, hold it open for everyone. Do know that there is evil in this world and you can't control it. What you can control are your thoughts and actions, so make them positive for others. You want to make this world better, right? Consciously think through every decision you make and ask, "Will this benefit me or someone else?" Many of the great leaders of today find ways to give back or take care of the people who believed in them during their rise to the top. Towards the end of the last millennium, Bill Gates and a couple of other ultra-rich people came together to make the Giving Pledge. It was a commitment to donate a significant percentage of their resources to charitable courses.

This is the mindset of successful people. We should constantly seek to help other people and make them happier.

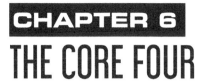
THE CORE FOUR

"The world breaks everyone, and afterward,
some are strong at the broken places."
– Ernest Hemingway

One of the most important concepts in life is finding balance in all of your core values. These core values should include living with a purpose, being healthy, serving others, and loving yourself. If a balance is not struck among these core values, our brains may begin to function counterproductively. Activities will only make us brainless for a certain period; they stimulate and fill the void of whatever it is we cannot fill with peace. Rather than being busy and productive, we tend to be more preoccupied. Power your body and your mind to trust in God, following His path and plan.

First let's talk about living with a purpose. Place your hand over your heart; can you feel it? That is called purpose. You're alive for a reason so don't ever give up. What are you passionate about? What do you prioritize and how do you spend your days? Didn't Dr. Seuss say it best, "Don't cry because it's over. Smile because it happened." There is so much to be passionate about: faith, music, family, work, traveling, serving and so on. You need to periodically take a break from your regular routine and make time to pursue your passions. Of course, you should work hard at your job, it's what puts food on your table. But jobs don't last forever. You'll retire someday, or worse still, you may get laid off for whatever reasons. It's your passions that you'll have to fall back on. So you should devote some time to them now. However, there should be a note of caution. When you rely only on your passion to make you happy, you will soon find out that life is very unbalanced. Remember that there are plenty of people out there who have families, work, and travel. They find a way to balance this out, and when life gets chaotic they adjust. If work becomes your main priority, then your family life may struggle and vice versa. It may be a little tough trying to balance everything and pull it all together. But you've got to trust God for help. As long as you put in the effort, He will strengthen you and make everything work out just fine.

Continue to put in the work required to pursue your passion but remember to keep a balance. It won't be easy at times but results never come from being a lazy bone. Search for your purpose; for some it comes naturally and for others it requires some digging. Ask yourself some questions that will help you discover your passions in life. What do you want your career to look like? What is the life goal that drives you? Where do you find your happiness? These can be intense questions, so take time to process your answers.

I do believe that everyone has some sort of burning passion in their hearts to be something they think they can't obtain. There's always some kind of lofty goal or breathtaking achievement that seems beyond our reach, but deep down we really desire it. Unfortunately, doubts and negativity often stop us from even attempting our secret, top of the rank ambitions. We talk ourselves out of it and leave it only in our imagination. For me, writing a book used to be such a big dream. Yet, with my pill addiction and all the negativity in my life, it felt like I would never be able to pull it off. But you're finally reading the result of my deciding to take the bull by the horn and go for my dream. Whether or not I was going to be a successful writer did not matter to me. I was fired up, and I needed to tell this story because

I was fed up with myself for not trying to be a better person. I wanted to see others set ablaze with the passion to be something different, try something new, and become someone better. Everyone can tap into this potential with something as simple as effort. Start small, dream big, and just go for it. Don't spread yourself thin, focus on your one main thing. And remember to make this main thing, the main thing. If you want to lose weight, start with your diet and make sure you are strict on your eating habits. If it is exercise, make sure you thoroughly track in a journal each individual workout.

Most of our dreams seem too large to achieve. When we want to reach these dreams, the steps we take seem too big. This results in a fear of failure. Train the brain to reduce stress through small, consistent steps. What is one thing I can change in my life to reduce stress? What can I start spending ten minutes on today to bring me closer to my goal? Completing these small steps gives a sense of accomplishment and encourages you to keep going. When you are working on these small steps, remember to have a relentless approach. New Year's Resolutions do not work; you simply have not trained the brain for long enough to make a habit, and you will keep falling back on old patterns.

Chase those dreams! Some people are left with the difficulty of narrowing down their dream into one perfect obtainable life. I honestly have never felt as if I should be doing just one job or living in one place throughout my life. I found out quickly that I am a nomad after moving away and traveling all over. This is where you can take time to dream big and visualize your perfect obtainable life and research how to make it a reality. Life moves at such a fast pace we tend to start settling down in our 30s. Many people are not anywhere near where they want to be in life at 30 years old. I certainly had a lot of questions.

Our next topic is about our health. Consciously think through what you fuel your body with. How does your body feel after the food you eat? Or after what you drink? It should feel energized and revitalized. Of course, there are over 32,000 different diets and all of them have worked for different people at different times. It all boils down to figuring out what works for you. You should know that an apple is better than those curly fries from Arby's, and a soda provides absolutely no nutritional value whatsoever. The problem is that we live in such a fast-paced world that the common, and, to be honest, the easiest option is typically not a healthy one. In my hometown I can only think of a handful of locations that offer something of nutritious value for an on-the-go person like me. Better eating starts with being informed or disciplined, or a combination of both. Many think that the best way to stop something is just to go "cold turkey." Not literally eat cold turkey but completely cut off your bad habit right then and there. When you tell yourself, I will do it tomorrow, you won't. Why put off what you can do today?

How about exercise? Combining healthy eating with exercising will give you more positive energy and focus as well. Using a schedule for exercise is important. Blocking off periods of time to go walk or run, lift weights, or stretch is important for your health. Starting off your day with a run and a healthy breakfast can go a long way. Try out different times of the day with your exercise and do what works best for you and your schedule. Make sure this is a part of your schedule. Instead of just sitting and watching TV, add some exercise in, do some triceps dips with the end of your chair, stretch or do sit-ups, jumping jacks, even consider running or jogging, perhaps just on a spot if you don't feel ready for the outdoors. Get enough sleep every night too, since rest is extremely important.

A healthy diet can go a long way towards helping you live a better life too. Stay disciplined and have someone hold you accountable if you truly want to make a change in your diet. Water, fruits, and vegetables are vital parts of any diet; there is no argument against that. With the likes of greasy burgers, Starbucks Frappuccino's, endless television shows, and social media, we make a majority of our decisions on impulse or for comfort. Taking small steps, making minor changes, and following this pattern for just a few weeks creates a new habit. Making the conscious decision to eat an apple for breakfast or get to the gym three times a week can change your life. For some it could be meditating or praying every morning before you grab your phone, writing a daily journal or choosing to look at life's smallest opportunities with a smile. We all can change.

Create opportunities to help a friend, donate your time, money, or volunteer. This willingness to give should come from the heart. Being overjoyed when helping someone is one of the greatest feelings in the world. If love is the universal language, then take the time to learn it and speak it! Think back to a time where you helped someone out. Perhaps it was a time when you helped a friend move, you volunteered at the soup kitchen, donated some clothes or money, how did it make you feel? Mark 10:45, Jesus said, "For even the Son of Man did not come to be served, but to serve, and to give his life as a ransom for many." You may even discover a sense of purpose through serving others. And without giving up on the pursuit of your own life's goals, you may discover a new one!

Take some time to look through your current situation in life. Ask yourself whether or not you can make some changes to help benefit others. The answer is yes—it's always yes. We always have the opportunity to change a few things in life to help others succeed or get better, so why not change? I know it is not an easy thing to do, to become selfless and do whatever is necessary to help others over yourself. But the good news is that it's worth it. The fulfillment, inner peace, and sense of meaning and usefulness that comes with helping others is more than enough compensation for the effort you have to make. Proverbs 11:27, "A generous person will prosper, whoever refreshes others will be refreshed." I have seen way too many times in mine and others' lives that hard work and generosity always gets rewarded. It just comes down to patience, persistence, and faith. Choose the right thing every day, find a way to help others, be honest, and know that your time will come sooner than later. Our society has turned more towards instant gratification. We all want to be happy, of course, but life is not easy. Most of what people choose to do in life is a temporary release from an emotion that causes the burden.

Finding contentment is not easy. Positive people always see opportunity in everything and everyone. They constantly seek adventure and have more questions than answers. Rarely are they satisfied with the results. They want more and desire better outcomes. What matters here is to live a life with which you are satisfied. Although life is unpredictable, you'll be happier if you have the knowledge that you're headed in the right direction. Stay focused, remember that each day will bring about new challenges and life may not go according to plan. Slow down and focus on the little things that bring happiness.

We live in a beautiful world! You can find happiness in something so simple. Take time to find peace, a bath or dinner by candlelight, meditate, pray and have some quiet time for yourself, put on a vinyl record, read a book, go for a walk and look at God's creation. When we find contentment, we will see the brilliance in God's plan to provide the happiness required to live a fulfilling life. There really is only one place to find true happiness, and that is within. Have you taken some time to smile when looking at your own reflection? Does your doubt outweigh your confidence? How can you find ways to be passionate yet content? Be satisfied with who you are and what you are doing in life and your mind will be at ease.

Most of us, including myself for a long time, think of meditation or silent time as a sign of weakness or "not a good fit." Whether this is because of our stubbornness, and for guys even testosterone, we close our minds off to any adventure that tends to expose us to the discomfort of the unknown. Even if it has been scientifically proven to promote health and reduce stress, we as humans just say no. If you have paid any attention throughout the Gospels in the Bible, you've seen that Jesus spent time every day in solitude and silence. He withdrew from people to pray and be alone with the Father. Jesus invites us to join him in this peace as well. So, if you think solitude and alone time isn't important, remember that Jesus made this one of his biggest priorities, and he turned out all right.

Another important habit is listening to music that causes your brain to reflect or energize. For some it may be jazz, classical, folk, country, pop, who knows, but consider music to be an amazing inspiration in your life. Be open to how it influences our attitudes and mindset. Playing or learning how to play an instrument can be extremely therapeutic as well. You can learn an immense amount about yourself through music. Music takes you to places within your mind that you never knew existed. Throughout the entire process of writing this book, I have had music on, and I can't reiterate enough how influential music is to the soul.

How can we show love to ourselves? Have a glass of wine, go shopping, go to a ball game, or take a walk in the woods, all by yourself. Think of a regular date, what would you do if you were taking, say, your girlfriend or boyfriend out? Well do that for yourself. Take time to learn, create, build, and discover new ways of thinking and doing. Slow down, close your eyes, and take a deep breath. Learn to appreciate who you are and what makes you special. When you start loving yourself more and more, everything in your life tends to improve. Your relationships blossom, you feel better, you realize that all of these simplistic changes in your life have the most profound impact on your mood. For many who struggle with loving themselves, remember that love is the glue that holds the entire world together.

Love is a deep connection to the universe; an intense appreciation of what God made us to be.

CHAPTER 7
FIND HAPPINESS AND EXPRESS JOY

"Happiness is when what you think, what you say,
and what you do are in harmony."
– Mahatma Gandhi.

The difficulty does not lie in trying, rather it is in sustaining the battle, whether it be internally in our hearts or brain, or externally through sources of advertisements or other social pressures. We constantly want to obtain happiness in a hasty fashion. Yet, life will not bend its rules just because our generation and age has chosen to take the fast lane. Good things, if they'll last, require consistent effort, persistence, and discipline. There is no magic wand to wave to create the perfect job or relationship— you get out of it what you give.

I have to reiterate a point about instant gratification and how it is not real. Block that fake reality out of your mind. Work hard, set goals, and know that it takes time to achieve them. It may not be six months or a year; it could be three years or even 10. It is a blessing to be alive, to be healthy, and to be able to walk, eat, breathe, and talk. Start off by being more thankful for what you have, because humility is very special.

Take some time to reflect on those key moments where you had your "aha" moment. Maybe it was when you felt like you really figured out how to be joyful or happy or even content. I doubt it was when you were texting or looking at pictures of cute dogs. This life is short, and many people just miss the point. We float along until the day we say goodbye to the people and universe that we hope we made an impact on. Put the device down, live in the now. Get out of your comfort zone and find a way to challenge yourself and the people around you. Deciding that this is who I am and what I want to be should not be embarrassing, because at the end of your life no one will care at all. You will only be able to reflect on who you were, how you treated others, and what type of impact you made on the world.

Think about what might happen if you can obtain this primary skill of selflessness early in life, and what you could then become. When you are selfless, an impact is made. Start with this question: Are you doing enough for the people who have influence on your life? Are you making sure they are on the right path and not your path? Everyone has their own journey that they create in life, but they need guidance and positive influences to help. The challenge is finding ways to become more selfless for people who are constantly focused on their image or happiness. It may take years or decades to get to the breakthrough point, so be patient. Don't spend all your time looking for happiness. You will end up missing joy.

I have asked a lot of questions so far, so let's take some time to reflect on what is absolutely necessary to start living a joyful life. Wisdom, balance, and patience. Start and end each day on a positive note. Connect with friends and family, be vulnerable. Exercise, volunteer, dance, set goals, meditate. Continue to seek what brings you happiness, surround yourself with whatever that may be and soon you will be full of joy. Patience is key to being content and knowing that you are not in control of what ultimately comes your way in life.

You need to be comfortable with the idea of not being in control, be it in your next relationship, job, or city. You may be able to take precautionary measures and try to be prepared, but I am sorry to break it to you, you are not in control, so accept that. Focus on getting wisdom above all else, for she is a beautiful source of life. To know patience is rare, it's unfamiliar, and many also see it as not being worth it either. The reason for this is not far-fetched; short term happiness and patience are often at odds with each other. It's difficult to choose to ride storms out and just hang on and see what life has in store for us. But guess what? Patience is actually a key requirement for living a fulfilled life.

I find myself asking the question, what is God up to? This curiosity draws me closer because I want to give all of my trust to His plan. Patience does not work by trusting in your own plans; rather, it is depending on God's plan, and He will reveal everything in His own time. Being patient in making decisions helps us to avoid committing sin. With patience, the focus shifts towards not engaging in our sinful nature, and we make better decisions. Suffering is patience. No one wants to suffer, but perseverance through suffering always bears fruit. If there is any primary skill in life that you should strive to acquire, let it be patience.

There is no denying that we all go through tough times in life. And this is the more reason why we need to learn patience. Also, being a patient person attracts selfless people into your life. These people will help you to get back on track whenever you begin to get anxious and lose your cool. Again, it may sound counterintuitive, but despite the uncertainty of life, it's still important to set goals and stick to them. And even in achieving our goals, patience is similarly important in sticking to the path and being eventually successful. This process tests patience, but the payoff is the greatest feeling you could ever experience!

As we know, life is not easy. We all want to do well and be good to those around us, but it just isn't that simple. We tend to lean on the notion of serving our own desires first, which then turns into a pattern and ultimately controls our thinking and decision making. If you are constantly worrying about what is next in life, then you are taking the potential joy out of today. The stress from wanting instant gratification will eventually eat you alive. Focus on the present, what you can do now and today that will leave you with the feeling of accomplishment. All journeys start somewhere. Maybe today is where you start over.

Now, you probably think at this point that you have to follow a completely strict schedule in order to maintain some sort of happiness, and that is not what I'm trying to portray. I am simply trying to push you towards a well-disciplined, selfless, and content approach with who you are and what you have in life. There is so much negativity in this world. The principles in this book may not work for you but find what does. These principles you follow should bring you enough happiness to fill the black hole that most people never figure out.

Here's a simple exercise to help set you on your path to finding joy in your life. Think about all the people around you, who would you consider the happiest? What do you think is responsible for them being so happy? If you can figure out the answer to that second question, fine! Go on and try to replicate it in your own life. However, if you think you don't know exactly why they're happy, then you'll have to take an important step and ask them. Yes! You read that right, walk right up to them and ask them how they manage to be so happy. No one is an island, we need other people to help us on the journey to happiness and self-improvement. When people realize that you're humble enough to ask questions and learn from them, they'll be willing to help you and push you forward.

I will continue to reiterate self-reflection and how important it is. This is essentially the same thing as taking your spiritual or emotional temperature. When you take the time to be mindful of your feelings, you can begin to understand the inner workings of yourself. Rather than staring at the ceiling, get up and start doing. Start to cross off your to-do list. Give no excuses, do not blame others, and embrace that change will always be challenging. Growth does not come without challenges.

Imagine being able to train our minds to remove the negative energy around us and build on the positives. We essentially would become what we feel, and that would be joyful. Take some time for yourself, cook a nice meal, go to the gym, listen to music, or call a friend. When the next sleepless night comes, rather than reaching for your cell phone, why not take a few minutes to reflect on who you are or even what you want to become? We must continue to reflect and be in tune with the world around us. For me, there will never be a car, house, vacation, or any other materialistic thing that could bring me more joy than loving myself. This starts with knowing I have a Father in Heaven who sacrificed his son, so I could have everything.

Before you work on pushing yourself, let's take time to think, really think about when you were full of joy. Why was this such a joyous time? Was it the people you were surrounded by? Was it the activity or place? Maybe, hopefully that time is right now and you're living in it! Take some time to reflect on that point in your life, smile, and laugh and enjoy what that moment feels or felt like all over again.

CHAPTER 8

TO BECOME ORDINARY OR THE RISK TAKER

"Too many of us are not living our dreams because
we are living our fears."
– Les Brown

As stated before, I had broken my collarbone playing soccer a few years ago but I was ready to start playing again. One summer day in San Antonio, Texas, I was playing soccer with my recreational team. I was dribbling the ball just outside of the goalie box when all of a sudden, I was smacked into by another opponent. I had felt the exact same pain that I did with the previous broken collarbone. I knew what was next, and I was not happy at all. The beauty of this story was what came from the second broken collarbone.

Surgery was imminent, but this time I had a different opportunity to take a risk for my healthcare career. I remember going into the pre-op surgery room and thinking this would be a wonderful time to make a sales pitch to my doctor to use me as a preferred provider for his patients. I remember laughing about it at first but knew that I probably wouldn't even remember asking for the business after the pain medications took effect and I was in surgery. I knew that if I never asked, I would have regretted it and most likely never had another opportunity. And little did I know that when I took the initiative and made my sales pitch with my brochures and business cards, the doctor was impressed and ultimately gave me an opportunity to be the home health provider for his patients. This relationship grew and ended up being one of the most important cornerstones for my business in healthcare.

The focus on that day of surgery was never intended to be on me getting answers about how the surgery would be performed or what rehab looked like. My mind was focused on getting business whether I failed or not. Taking risks has and always will be in my blood. I do not intend to live a comfortable life. This is not a recommendation for those who have accepted their lot in life or do enjoy the comfort of what their current situation is. There is absolutely nothing wrong with either path, but I do believe that everyone should at least ask themselves these questions. Am I happy with my comfortable life? Should I take more risks? Or should I find more comfort in my life, and take less risk?

While it's true that there's no guarantee for seeing tomorrow, this should not stop you from thinking about the future and preparing for it. We look up to God in faith to bring us hope for better days. As Christians, we know that ultimately following His path will bring us through tough times. There have been moments in my life when I have felt as if I was suffocating and could not get through my situation. However, the hope I had for better days ultimately released the tension, gave me the motivation to get out of bed and try my best to be a better person for everyone. I have been through plenty of pain and struggle. Just like me, you can come out stronger after fighting through the valley.

Continually seeking new ways to improve your mind will enhance your life. Trying out new foods, places, and activities causes the brain to react in unfamiliar ways, thus expanding your capacity. When I was living in a primarily Hispanic culture in Texas, I learned so much about family and culture. It opened my eyes to a new light of connection. The wealth of knowledge I learned from traveling and living in different areas of the U.S.A. has impacted me so much. I hadn't realized it at that time, but that experience showed me the importance of connection and community.

Do you live an exciting life? Or like most people, do you find most of your days to be routine? There seems to be a gap between fulfillment and hope. Many people are quick to lose hope when dreams are shattered. Although God promises fulfillment that cannot be found anywhere else, our negativity still finds ways to overpower hope.

On the other hand, routine can be great for most people. Eat, sleep, work, and repeat. Were we brought into this world to just be okay with routine? If you took the time to read this book knowing it was going to challenge your thinking, then your answer is probably no. Start by taking some alone time. Take a half hour in the morning and meditate, pray, or just sit in silence and think about what you are going to accomplish for that day. What are your goals for the day? Prioritizing what you do in life will not only lead you to be more successful, but it will fill some of that void with which you put empty and useless nonsense. Put away the phone!

There is true beauty in being able to appreciate the ordinary things in life. Although it may at times feel mundane and quite repetitive, would you risk throwing it all away for something or someone else? What I mean by 'ordinary' are things like fatherhood, 8-5 jobs, or your evening routine of dinner and TV. Although I do believe we were put on this earth to be unique and adventurous, there seems to be no greater joy than being a parent. And who says being a father or mother is ordinary anyway? When you question if this ordinary lifestyle is for you, remember you are probably doing it with people you love, and there is nothing that can be more fulfilling than making efforts to take care of people you love. No matter what path you choose in this life, remember to never regret, and always smile.

Many of us continually sulk on the difficulties in life and rarely look at the positives. As many know, the best things in life are free but they can also be quite complex. Sometimes they require some serious work, like relationships, being a parent, a boss, an athlete, or a Christian.

To make something out of nothing is quite a surreal feeling. I tried so many different career paths at which I failed, which ultimately led me to telling my story, thus creating a new passion and hopefully a successful career. It took me years to get to this point, but there really is no reason to be embarrassed about anything anymore.

This is what I want more of the people around me to be like: vulnerable and willing to admit their flaws or struggles. I think it is a natural tendency for humans to want to help others or change themselves. We just continue to disregard these changes because it is too inconvenient or difficult. I believe all of this starts with attitude. Deciding to be positive no matter the circumstance or situation can go a long way. No one will ever want to be around negativity for too long. At the end of your life you probably would not want people to remember you for your grumpiness, right? Unfortunately, there is so much that's beyond your control, but your attitude plays a huge role in dealing with situations like these.

Being contrarian in life is similar to being a risk taker. When you put yourself out there and decide to be brave, it often leads to more fruitful relationships and deeper connections with people. Having the same conversation about the weather, work, and sports, or how your weekend was, is in itself boring, repetitive, and unproductive at times. Dig deeper with people, get more personable and find out who they are or what they want to be. Become the person who welcomes others in and ask for people to share their feelings and experiences with you. This is another great example of how to overcome loneliness as well.

Most people feel uncomfortable sharing feelings or expressing themselves freely with no regard to the reaction. Risk taking is almost unorthodox in society, and some people feel as if change is bad, so they stick to their course without even attempting to become something they strive for. Living in fear can be a powerful thing, and I am here to tell you that no one cares. An opinion someone has of you does not ultimately matter. If you believe in yourself, then you have accomplished one of the hardest tasks in life. Be willing to fail because nearly 80% of the millionaires in this world have failed multiple times, filed for bankruptcy, were homeless, and so on. Be that risk taker, gamble on yourself if you truly want to change your life. Draw up a plan for your course of action, take time to talk with friends and family about it, pray and seek answers.

To keep up with the world you must constantly be learning. Reading more books than your colleagues, learning new and innovative ways to improve, trying out new hobbies or activities to learn more about your brain. Most people travel the common road, the more familiar life that is not as challenging but is predictable and monogamous. Maybe this is what works for you, or maybe you worked so hard to get to the point where you enjoy this consistent day to day operation. Just remember to find what works and stick with it.

The ultimate goal of pushing through unchartered territories should be to create kindness and love for others. It may seem selfish to take a risk on something to create a better life for yourself, but then turning this transformation into something beautiful can happen for others.

The truth is that following God's plan for my life made everything fall into place so perfectly. Life becomes more about what time I could spend helping others and the impact I could make in their lives. We should reinvent ourselves, restructure our lives, and reenergize the people around us. Become a light for anyone and everyone. Begin feeling the raw emotions associated with living a real and purposeful life. Throw out old ways of thinking, biases, and stubbornness. Work on being a better listener, be honest about your own flaws, and be open with everyone. This will lead to stronger and deeper relationships.

I have had my fair share of failure in my life, an incredible amount. I first took a shot at being a school teacher. I had taken all the courses and prepared for the test, but I failed on the first try and gave up on that dream. Next, I wanted to be a realtor in Texas. I was inspired to become something I was very passionate about. I took all the courses in just under four months and prepared for the test. I only passed one of the two tests and then found out shortly after I would be moving away from Texas. I lost the motivation to try again due to these circumstances, so I just gave up and moved on. I also had two different businesses, one focused on photography and graphic design and the other a stock trading venture. Both had their successes, but ultimately ended up in failure.

So, I continued to ask myself, am I seeking my passion, or do I already know what it is? Many people find themselves settling for whatever is easy or comfortable. Many find their career path early on, take the first job out of high school or college, and just go with the flow. The question that needs to be answered is this: Are you passionate about your work? Are there any opportunities to pursue your passions outside of your normal job? I found out in the long run that I was very passionate about serving others, connecting and improving relationships.

Are you excited about waking up every day to your current line of work?

Or is it the constant struggle, day to day kind of life that is causing chaos? The grind can be tough, finding what you love, making it become your life. You can use several routes to find this out. Trying various jobs, experimenting with different groups or networks, or for the more fortunate, following a calling from your childhood or teenage years, among others.

Doing more with less. The phrase *doing more with less* has become somewhat of a battle cry for many businesses and organizations across the world. But not only is this important in business, it can be an interesting metaphor for change within ourselves. Why is it so hard to raise the bar on our own goals and expectations by doing more with less? It does not mean more hours at work or in the gym, it is all about the concept of being smarter and prioritizing our time. The current set up of our society, with Netflix and social media, allows for a lot of time getting wasted without even being noticed. Many people wake up with the intention to have a great day and get things done. But suddenly, it's 9pm and you realize you've not touched your to-do list, and you're refreshing Instagram for the 167th time that day. Your life doesn't have to continue being like this. I've heard people complain that we need more than 24 hours in a day. But that's wrong. 24 hours are actually more than enough. The actual problem is what we do with the time. By learning to maximize and fully utilize our resources, most importantly time, we can achieve far more and create the kind of life we always wanted.

Find someone who forces you to grow in aspects of life you think you don't need. Learn about odds and ends that are outside your usual circle, something different from what you learnt in college, something unrelated to what you do for a living at work. Becoming a generalist or a polymath used to be frowned upon, but many leaders including Bill Gates, Warren Buffett, Elon Musk, Larry Page, and Jeff Bezos are polymaths. They may be great leaders in business, but they continually seek new ways to improve and learn. We need these opposites in our lives to enhance our growth and open our minds to new possibilities. Learn to love all and be kind to everyone you meet.

When we set preconceived notions about people, our minds have already shifted towards a negative feeling. Personally, I have been at fault concerning this in the past, but I'd like to talk about a relationship that developed after starting off on the wrong foot.

One of my best friends and I were raised in completely different environments. He was out living on his own at an early age, going to school and working full time to help pay his bills. Sleeping on floors at times, or wherever he could find a bed, was not easy for him.

I was raised with all the support I needed and was able to live in a comfortable home without much financial stress. There were very few obstacles for me in my young adult life as well.

But one day, he and I met on a basketball court at the local YMCA in Fort Wayne, Indiana. We certainly did not get along well in the beginning, as we were constantly trying to be the best through competition. We butted heads on and off the court, and there was very little respect for one another at this point in our lives. I was young at the time, but I certainly did not take the chance to get to know him very well.

One day everything changed. He was brought on to work with me at our local hardware store called McCord's Do It Best. We were essentially forced to learn how to coexist as coworkers. We were opposites when it came to our sports teams as well. I was a Michigan fan, and he was a diehard Notre Dame fan. I knew that God had a plan of teaching me yet another valuable lesson here. As time went by we learned that although we had all of these differences, we had a lot of respect for each other.

His hard work mentality pushed me to do better at my job, and I would like to believe my faith in God taught him some valuable lessons along the way as well. This relationship is a living example of the power of Christ. Later, we were fortunate enough to work together again at a healthcare company. And as both of us began working the long hours and life adjusted, I made the drastic decision to move away to Texas. Although I enjoyed the job and where my career was heading, I felt that God was leading me elsewhere. Matt went ahead and took over my job when I moved. And just as expected, he did very well, received a promotion, and became one of the most successful sales associates in the entire company nationwide. These stories of starting from nothing and becoming a leader are out there. I was able to witness this through Matt. His story continues to be a powerful motivator for me to become something much more.

I hope that these types of people are in your life, no matter who they are, what they look like, or what they believe. The powerful motivator types, although they may seem rare, you could just be looking in the wrong spot. Unfortunately, we see much of a different notion in society. Many individuals feel privileged, and we constantly boost them up no matter what. There was a specific group in my younger days called the untouchables. Why have we continued to put labels on groups? We are encouraging segregation and allowing more animosity toward others than ever before. The world needs more healthy debates with people who have minds open to listening to others. Love is a universal language, and that starts with listening regardless of whether you agree or disagree with whomever is talking.

CHAPTER 9
CAN LONELINESS BE A GIFT FROM GOD?

"If you could only sense how important you are to the lives of those you meet; how important you can be to the people you may never even dream of. There is something of yourself that you leave at every meeting with another person."
- Fred Rogers

I struggled with the meaning of this for quite some time. How can loneliness be a gift? Why does anyone have to be alone? God teaches us some amazing lessons through our loneliness. Many of us have experienced loneliness in all different situations in life. It may be in a large crowd of people, with friends or family, or even lying next to a spouse. There is also uncontrollable loneliness, such as how you feel after losing a loved one, sickness, a bad break up, a job loss, and so on. And when this hits us, we often feel some of the most excruciating pain that we have ever experienced. Is there a smart way to address this feeling?

In Luke 5:16 it says, "But Jesus often withdrew to lonely places and prayed." There is a foundation for some amazing growth in our loneliness. If Christ saw this as an opportunity for hope and strength, imagine what we as humans can do! This loneliness feeling that everyone experiences bleeds in my writing throughout this book. As painful as it was at times,

God showed me how incredibly powerful He is, and He gave me the most strength that I could have ever experienced in life.

I fought this loneliness just as many of us do. We take our loneliness and fill it with external sources of pleasure or comfort to numb the pain. Our busyness becomes the distraction from true growth as individuals. When we decide that this is the answer to our problems, the devil wins the battle. We even start to believe lies that we tell ourselves during our loneliness. These lies then make a significant impact on our overall mood and happiness. This approach is wrong, we shouldn't try to avoid loneliness or numb it away. It's something we should embrace and see as a genuine source of growth. You may be convinced that no one at all cares about you, rather than looking towards Christ for comfort and help. When I felt this loneliness becoming overbearing, I gave all I had to Him for help. I knew that this suffering would not last, and I knew that diving deeper would strengthen my faith. There is no superhuman out there who can do it all on his own. We all need someone to lean on at times, and the only truth is that God is the one.

Paul Banks once said, *"I'm sick of spending these lonely nights training myself not to care."*

I battled with this quote for a long time. Spending what seemed like endless nights alone for years of my life. Rarely feeling comfortable being alone, yet also not willing to ask for help. After thinking about this quote for a long time, I knew that it was my fault. This was not only a true wakeup call for myself, but one of the biggest inspirations behind this book. We need to be comfortable alone, but we also need to know when to ask for help. The battle I faced was not being able to admit I felt lonely when honestly, I felt completely alone. God was not at the forefront anymore, but I knew deep down that He was always watching over me. As the pain of loneliness grew and my happiness withered, everything fell apart. Deep down there was no question about how much I had screwed up my life. I was just too stubborn to accept it. However, that day on Mount Cutler changed my life. Everything began to feel different. I no longer felt alone. I knew that God had taught me so many valuable lessons and in turn opened my heart to writing this book. How can we, as a society find ways to reach people who feel like this? I think it tracks back to being attentive and genuinely caring about others. If we don't try to reach out to people, we won't know if they're sad or lonely. Without faith, my family and friends, I would not be on this earth right now.

Just think about what Christ endured to free us from our sins. Now take the focus away from yourself for a second and imagine His suffering. Because if anyone understands your feeling of loneliness or pain, it is Jesus and Him alone. He's been there. Up on that cross with his most trusted disciples and friends either running away from him or watching him helplessly. Even God, his father, looked away, Jesus was completely alone on that cross. His only companions on that cross were pain, betrayal, and sadness. Therefore, when you want to fill the void of loneliness, take time to talk to God. This is exactly what He wants your relationship to be about. Talking, asking, and even requesting opportunities to happen in your life. How about what Jabez said in 1 Chronicles 4:10: "Jabez cried out to the God of Israel, 'Oh, that you would bless me and enlarge my territory! Let your hand be with me and keep me from harm so that I will be free from pain.' And God granted his request." How simple is that? If He wants you to lean on him during your loneliness, just imagine what the result will be when you put your complete trust in Him to fix your loneliness. How can you ever get what you want without asking? If you just sit back and continue to complain about your situation, you will never get answers. Just like in every other lesson I am trying to teach in this book, hard work and consistency are required. One simple prayer for a cure to loneliness or pain perhaps will not yield the result you want. Once you give yourself completely over to Him and allow Him to work in and through you, then you will start to see progress.

Another interesting way to look at loneliness as a positive is in seeing what it does for our own personal growth. We discover more about ourselves, what interests us, and we start improving our lives in order to fill the void of this lonely feeling. If you can't start loving yourself first, you will never be able to receive love or give love to others. Withdrawing to be alone is not necessarily a bad thing. In fact, it can be a true blessing. This loneliness we experience exposes a lot of our sinful nature and how we can improve rather than dwell in it. When we choose to use this time to draw nearer to God and hear what He has to say, we become more reliant on his teachings. Our trust and hope grow as well as our faith. The teachings are invaluable. When we trust in the Lord to fix our loneliness, He gives us more for which to be thankful. We all are sinners, and when we reflect in this alone time, we can begin to take notice of what we want and need to change to grow.

What do you think God is incapable of doing? If you have an answer other than nothing to this question, then you have found a good starting point to fix your problems. This potentially can be one of the greatest turning points in your life as well. When you surrender to the Lord, you are also at the beginning of obedience. God simply wants us to follow His plan, because no matter what your argument is, His plan is better.

Rick Warren puts it perfectly, *"God wants you to decide in advance, trusting him and believing that His will is the best plan for your life."*

That word surrender should not deter you from becoming who you want to be. Surrendering allows God to be in control and our fears are only focused on disappointing our Father. This surrendering will strengthen your adaptability as well, and it is part of the growth mindset too. Is there anything that you truly believe is impossible? Because the truth is, "Jesus looked at them and said, 'With man this is impossible, but with God all things are possible." (Matthew 19:26) That statement alone is so incredibly powerful!

When our will to overcome and persevere in the darkest days is weak, we must find ways to press on. Sometimes it even requires a self-pep talk, a good cry, a run on the treadmill, or alone time. All of these things may seem inane or even childish, but they can be the boost you need to keep holding on. Life is not meant to be lived alone, and our loneliness should always be filled with something or someone of value.

Always count your blessings, because we often forget to reflect on them and we should do it more often. When we get trapped in a negative thought process, we feel the loneliness become the cloud over our heads even on sunny days. Just like fixing any problem powered by negativity, we need to establish coping mechanisms to deal with the emptiness feelings too. Find someone to reach out to; if you don't have any family then consider a therapist, as there is no shame in that. When you feel lonely, consider helping others, because volunteering your time for others is extremely beneficial for your loneliness as well as your mental health. And remember, God is always there for you. He wants to listen, and He encourages you to speak to Him.

STORY OF JONAH

Jonah was from Israel. The word of the Lord came to Jonah, directing him to go to Nineveh in the North and tell them the good news about Him. God said, "Tell the people that if they don't stop sinning I will smite them all!" Jonah was scared about this proposition from God and thought it would be better to just run away. Thinking he could outsmart God, he hopped on a boat and headed to Spain. On the way to Tarshish, a terrible storm popped up in the sea. Jonah was below deck at the time, asleep while all the sailors were scared for their lives. These sailors asked Jonah to pray to his God to save them. They began throwing their luggage off board and Jonah felt as if he was at fault as well. He told them he was the problem and that they would be fine as soon as he was taken out. So, he was hurled off the boat too. God had arranged for Jonah to not die here in the water, so a giant fish came and swallowed Jonah but did not chew him up into little bits and pieces. Jonah ended up living in this giant fish for three days. He had some time while sitting in the belly of this fish to think about his life and what he was doing with it. He asked God for help and vowed to make good. I'd like to point out that it was the period of loneliness within the fish's belly that brought Jonah back to his senses and got him back on track. This giant fish ended up puking Jonah up onto the shore, back where he started in the North.

Jonah knew that God intended for this to happen and that this time he needed to go tell the people that God was going to smite them because they were being so sinful. Although the people did not firmly believe in the same God that Jonah did, they felt nervous and prayed to the Lord asking Him to not kill them. They all fasted to show God how sorry they were for sinning so much and being so violent. After God saw them turn from their evil ways, he did not bring the destruction on them that he had once threatened.

You would think at this point that Jonah would be happy, but no, he was very sad. He said, "Now, LORD, take away my life, for it is better for me to die than to live." (Jonah 4:3)But the LORD replied, "Is it right for you to be angry?" (Jonah 4:4) Jonah then went out to make some shelter just east of the city. God helped grow a vine over Jonah's head to provide shade and comfort for him. Jonah was now happy! And then God provided a worm who came and ate the vine, and the tree died. Jonah became faint and said again that he wanted to die. God's illustration was simple. Without tending to the plant and helping it grow, it can wither and die overnight. Just like the 120,000 people who needed God, Jonah was only thinking of himself.

CHAPTER 10
THE NEW YOU

*"Every day, you reinvent yourself. You're always in motion.
But you decide every day: forward or backward."*
– James Altucher.

I remember hearing the train behind my parent's house every morning at 6am and every night at 9:30pm when I was a kid growing up. I loved hearing the horn and always wished I would have become a conductor when I got older. Well, that dream left me once I realized how lonely I would have been. Traveling between different locations, only communicating with the crew, probably never being able to settle down in one spot. The ironic thing is, when I moved away at 23 years old, I told myself I would never be back to hear that train again. And right before my 31st birthday, I was back. I soon remembered how much of an impact that train noise made on me as a child, and how as an adult it was completely different.

I had dreams as a child, and the train symbolized hope. In my adult life, the train symbolized faith. I followed a terrible routine of negative talk when I first moved back. I lost a partner, a dog, a family, a city, most of my possessions, and many friends. I certainly couldn't get out of the funk of the negativity for quite a while. The darkness seemed to engulf me, and my mood sank really low. This time though I remembered my trust in the Lord, and my faith gave me hope again. I knew I would have to suffer plenty of consequences for my mistakes. I knew that the trials I was about to face were going to be difficult and at times feel impossible to surmount. My brain needed to be trained to block out the negative and focus on my faith. Everything was going to be fine, I just needed to get the crap kicked out of me and battle, never stop the fight. I trusted through the tears and the anger. I told myself plenty of times I couldn't do it, but deep down there was never going to be any quit.

The stories I have read about people making big positive changes continue to be a huge encouragement for me to keep going and never stop evolving. So let me ask again, what can we do right now, today, this very minute to change our lives for the better of everyone, including ourselves? Write it down on your hand, in your journal, send it in an email to yourself, to your best friend, dad or mom, whomever, this process will solidify it; take it from the realm of being just an idea to a real entity.

I can tell you first and foremost that my situation was not even close to how bad other people have it. I actually had it made. I was able to come home to a house and be welcomed by my parents. Good friends of mine found me a great job to get me back on my feet within a few weeks. I was humbled so fast. Although I had lost a majority of my life in a matter of days, I had what many don't get in life: a second chance. I was not going to let my past failures control my future.

I began to lay out my goals. I began writing and journaling everything. It became therapeutic. I knew that the only way to get through a rut was to do the ugly and dirty work necessary to survive. Work hard, quit all of my bad habits, and develop new and productive routines. What began with simple tasks like reading the Bible and praying for 30 minutes before I got up, turned into working out four to five times a week and meditating every morning before I went to work. The hard work was ahead of me every day, but as I began the process, everything became more natural and I knew I was on the right path.

My mood had changed; my outlook on life changed. I did not feel like I was doing much to make me happy, but I was doing all of the right things. It took me over four months of grinding to realize that I was making progress. I was so sad throughout those first four months that I honestly felt like giving up several times. Dark, gloomy days in Indiana sitting behind a computer desk or with my pen and paper are not the most pleasant experiences in the world. You can bet I was determined to do what I felt was going to save my life. I would pop on a record, typically Frank Sinatra, grab a glass of wine, light a candle, and just write. I found a new therapy, and I never thought it would end up saving my life.

"Writing--and this is the big secret--wants to be written. Writing loves a writer the way God loves a true devotee. Writing will fill your heart if you let it. It will fill your pages and help to fill your life."
- Julia Cameron

One of my favorite lines from a song is, "From the ashes a new life is born." Take the opportunity when you hit your low to realize that you are so close to an unbelievable life ahead of you. I won't try to delude you, it's not easy! When you're down in the pit of depression, it feels like there's no light in sight and there can be no way out. But you have to struggle to keep hope alive within you. Time heals, faith seals, God reveals. Trust the process. You will continue to have setbacks and times of utter disappointment, but do not let your brain overtake your heart because all of this pain is temporary! There will be a point in your life where you reach the limit of misery and disarray you can put up with to maintain happiness. You won't necessarily know this limit or identify it, but once you reach it, the only option is to deal with it. This goes back to the argument about being proactive vs. reactive. It's much easier to do the right thing from the start. If this is not the case, remember that you canalways turn it around. Just remember to always love yourself, no matter what. And don't ever give up; don't even let that be an option.

In life people will be mean to you, speak negatively about you, and they will wrong you. These moments will test you as an individual. You have two options here. The low road, or the high road. Bitterness is not pretty on you, it does not befit you. And ugliness is not the answer either. When you take the high road you should feel proud about how you reacted in a certain situation. This will be a big challenge when trying situations occur. Most have used revenge as therapy because releasing anger feels great, right? Of course, we all know anger works as a short-term solution just as drug use, sex, or alcohol are short-term releases from anxiety or everyday stresses in life. When you wrong someone, remember, ask for forgiveness and take the necessary steps to fix the problem you created. The people who want you in their life will forgive and forget. Just make sure you fix your issues and never stop working on being a better person for everyone around you.

Investing in your future starts with prioritizing your life. Set goals and follow through. Listen to advice from people who want you to succeed rather than listening to the negative people who say you're being too risky or that isn't smart. You have predetermined that this is what you want in life and you are going to accomplish it no matter what, so why should a person's negative thoughts control you? I had made up my mind quickly when I got back that I was not going to settle for a normal job and a normal life. I started to research everything in my life that ever interested me as a job. From missionary work to traveling as a nurse or starting another small business, I opened my mind to endless possibilities, which gave me more and more hope every day. This all started with goal setting and prioritizing important activities over fun.

How can we begin the work of creating a new future? Take the next step by writing down five dreams or goals. These can be anything—don't limit yourself! My five dreams were to help build a hospital, become a recognized writer, visit India, speak on a stage in front of thousands of people, and go to a soccer game in Manchester. Quite a variety, but you get the idea. Dream big! Focusing on dreams, goals, or a bucket list will increase dopamine. Positive thoughts will soon turn into positive actions. Just continue to focus on the end goal with patience, persistence, and relentlessness. Developing good habits changes everything and thinking positively and being confident can go a long way in life.

Make a daily schedule for what you want to prioritize in life. If you want to focus on eating better, then write down meal plans for the week and stick to it. If your focus is on work, find ways to be efficient with your time in meetings, have questions ready, or set a goal for what you want to achieve each single day. Just remember, this takes time. You will fail at times; you will have setbacks. You will repeat old behaviors and wonder why you are getting the same results.

Everyone should have a life goals or bucket list. Take at least 30-60 minutes to create this list and try to come up with several different ideas. Mine was composed of mostly places I wanted to travel to, with some activities as well. Don't limit yourself; write down whatever comes to your mind. Be ambitious, courageous, and even write down what you think may be unattainable. You may think about getting your pilots license or learning a different language; whatever you desire, put it in writing. We all have a hunger for something. None of us were born without it.

Many of us may write down this list of goals and think that most are just impossible and unrealistic. Why is that? Are you really scared of failure or embarrassment even? "Claim your ghost" is a line that has always stuck with me. What is it that makes you feel trapped? Is there something that may even be haunting you?

Creating a new you requires some major changes. We as humans tend to do three different things with ourselves. We think and feel that we are this type of person, we present ourselves to others as a different person, and we want to become something totally different from both previous versions. How can we get to the point where we feel comfortable showing others our true self?

For me, that feeling of embarrassment and criticism weighed me down. God created us all with vastly different minds, and we should use them to discover ourselves more. When you sit down and write out how you identify yourself, are you portraying yourself as a different person to others? If so, why? I have been guilty of this. Most people I met when I was younger said I was cocky, arrogant, or stubborn. I felt that I was confident, but I also did not realize that I was not humbly confident. I boasted way too much about my athletic ability or sales skills. Someone once made that very clear to me, I knew I needed to change. Doesn't 2 Corinthians 11:30 put it best? "If I must boast, I will boast of the things that show my weakness."

Thus, I ask myself, am I the same person when I am alone and another person when I'm around others? After a lot of hard work, I believe I am making strides but I'm nowhere near where I should be. Do you feel this way? Most of the help for me came from mentors and friends who called me out on my bull crap. Now with this book as a platform, I want to call you out on your bull crap too. No longer will there be time for excuses about why we cannot get better as individuals and as a society. I want to empower others to succeed, and I want the same in return.

The truth is that our society puts too much emphasis on independence and individual expression. We need others in order to succeed on our own journey, whatever that may be. Because to become the ideal person you strive to be, you must present yourself to others in the same way that you think and feel you are already. Whether you think you may be in an identity crisis or you feel lost, reevaluate with these three questions. Who am I? Who do others think I am? What do I want to become? Answers to these questions will provide you with a template of how to change to heal yourself and get better.

Let's now focus on how we can create this template for growth. Have you ever taken the time to just sit and write out your thoughts or feelings? This exercise will open your mind up and help you discover who you really are and what you enjoy.

When you first begin the journaling process, you may drift towards talking about your feelings or how angry you were with the waiter that served you at a restaurant. Whatever direction your free thinking flows on to paper, study and process it, and then decide if changes need to be made from what you observed. It is likely that you will have to make some big changes to fix your thinking process. The best idea here is to journal at different times for at least a few weeks. Even consider recording yourself on your phone and then listening at a later time. This idea slowly develops an awareness for how your brain works. Hopefully you discover some positives from the journaling that can help you progress. Many, including myself, use a similar system in work as well. Journaling about various conversations that you have with business partners or friends and family will show different tendencies as well. Maybe you will discover you react quite differently with certain people than you do with others, or even when you are alone. Becoming aware and developing a plan of action on how to improve is the goal with this type of journaling. Once again, be open minded and consider this practice. It could be the start of an amazing change!

And here's another great exercise that can help start the transition from selfish to selfless. Take small steps by writing down five things you are most grateful for in your life right before you go to sleep. Put this list somewhere that you will see every night. For me, I wrote down family, friends, God, health, and my job. After you make your list, start to focus on each individual one. There is so much to be thankful for in life, so take some time to smile on your five choices. This should certainly start to put life into perspective for you.

The process of becoming more selfless requires reflection. When you continue to think about the amazing parts of your life, your focus becomes positive. Of course, we still need to take care of ourselves, but the focus right now is on training the mind to think of others first. Taking a true assessment of how you fill your time up will show you what tendencies you have. Are you using all of your precious time for yourself? Or, are you making time to help others grow?

All of these different mindsets have causes and effects. Taking the posture of open mindedness, positive thinking, and helpful intentions allows us to become something greater than ourselves. We begin to evolve from a selfish to a selfless type. We can then see the impact that love has on others and what amazing love we will get in return. So don't just go part of the way, go all the way. Commit to change within yourself and help others around you.

People naturally gravitate towards happier people. It is almost by natural selection that we choose to surround ourselves with positive, hardworking, and happy people. This is all part of becoming positive as a whole, surrounding yourself with the right people, doing the right things, and being thankful for any and every opportunity you have in life. During your alone time, what exactly are you doing? Distracting yourself, or taking the time to be productive? Explore who you are more, find ways to be creative, write down your thoughts about your day or just about anything.

If all of these lessons I have learned in life can somehow impact just one person, then I know that God is working in them just like He is in me. Ever heard the saying about having an attitude of gratitude? When the focus begins with thinking about what we are thankful for, our minds react positively. Consider what makes you happy and focus on that. This is essential and critical to progress and getting rid of all the negativity. Life can throw us curveballs and cause us to take some drastic measures to fix problems or situations. Taking on these problems with a concerned or angry mind can cause even worse repercussions.

I remember hearing a phrase a while back: "embrace the suck." When you are going through tough times, sadness, anger, whatever it may be, embrace it and know that God will turn your life around. It is one of the toughest tasks to have a positive attitude during the rough times. I felt like I finally had turned a corner and was gaining momentum during my low point. And then suddenly, I had some major setbacks that took me back to square one. I got sick and tired of feeling so down I knew I had to just embrace whatever happened next. My car was then smashed twice in the same day, within the same hour, by two different drivers, and all my dad and I could do was laugh. God was definitely having fun at this point. I would continue to pray for a breakthrough every day, sometimes every hour. I knew this pain was temporary, but it was so deep and powerful. At times I just wanted to be alone, not be around anyone other than my music and my writing. I looked at this time as an opportunity to grow as a person, learn about my creative side, do something positive, and accomplish what I have been wanting to do for years. In fact, I started writing this book on Halloween in 2006 but took about eight years off in between. My brain had evolved quite a bit during this time, and I became more inspired than ever to write and write and write.

There was nothing that could stop me from finishing this book; it had to be done.

CONCLUSION

"Never stop. Never stop fighting. Never stop dreaming."
– Tom Hiddleston

Thank you for taking the time to read through this book.

Throughout the process of writing this book, I felt God's presence all around me. From the time on Mount Cutler, to the deer and the moon. In between the hard days and tough times, He was there. It was the most incredible experience I have ever had in my life. God woke me up. This awakening sparked a flame in my heart to write this story.

My hope is that it makes a real difference in your life for the better. Go hug your family or call a friend. Volunteer to work for a charity even if you don't have money to donate. Pack your bags and go on that safari vacation you've always dreamed of. And, most importantly, don't ever forget to show love; it could save someone's life. And whatever pain you are experiencing, perhaps it is loneliness, sadness, anger or regret, remember, it doesn't have to be like this.

Yesterday is history, tomorrow is a mystery, we only have today – let us begin!